NATUR. HAND CARE

HERBAL TREATMENTS AND SIMPLE TECHNIQUES FOR HEALTHY HANDS AND NAILS

NORMA PASEKOFF WEINBERG

STOREY BOOKS
Schoolhouse Road
Pownal, Vermont 05261

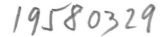

ACKNOWLEDGMENTS

I want to thank everyone who lent me a hand in this project: the reference librarians in Cape Cod and Boston public libraries; the Herb Society of America; the herbalists and other experts interviewed, who freely shared their time, energy, and wisdom; the reviewers, Robert Foley, Ila Hirsch, Michael Janson, M.D., Larry B. Meyerson, M.D., Lawrence A. Norton, M.D., and Nikolaus J. Smeh, for their patient advice; and my editors and the enthusiastic staff at Storey Books.

*The mission of Storey Communications is to serve
our customers by publishing practical information that encourages
personal independence in harmony with the environment.*

Edited by Deborah Balmuth, Pamela Lappies, and Nancy Ringer
Text design and production by Susan Bernier and Erin Lincourt
  (based on an original design by Carol Jessop, Black Trout Design)
Production assistance by Jennifer Jepson
Cover design by Carol Jessop, Black Trout Design
Cover illustration by Laura Tedeschi
Drawings by Kathy Bray and Laura Tedeschi, except pages 108 by Randy Mosher,
  150 by Alison Kolesar, and 204 by Beverly Duncan
Indexed by Hagerty & Holloway

Copyright © 1998 by Norma Pasekoff Weinberg

Printed in the United States by R.R. Donnelley
10 9 8 7 6 5 4 3 2 1

Library of Congress Cataloging-in-Publication Data

Weinberg, Norma Pasekoff
    Natural hand care / Norma Pasekoff Weinberg.
        p.   cm.
    Includes bibliographical references and index.
    ISBN 1-58017-053-6 (pb : alk. paper)
    1. Hand—Care and hygiene—Popular works.   2. Nails—Care and hygiene—Popular works.   3. Beauty, Personal.   4. Hand—Diseases—Alternative treatment—Popular works.
I. Title.
    RA776.5.W438   1998
    646.7'2—dc21   98-4409
                                                                            CIP

APPLAUSE FOR NATURAL HAND CARE

Natural Hand Care *is informative, a delight to read, and full of wonderful recipes and remedies. It's the most comprehensive book I've seen on the subject of hands. I loved it! A must for anyone who works with their hands.*

— Mary Bove, N.D., naturopathic doctor,
Brattleboro Naturopathic Clinic, Brattleboro, Vermont

If you have two hands and you want to keep them healthy, this book will be a valuable resource.

— Michael Janson, M.D., president, American College for Advancement in Medicine,
and author of *The Vitamin Revolution in Healthcare*

I found Natural Hand Care *entertaining and informative. This book empowers the reader to be the first line of defense in caring for their own hands. I can't wait to try some of the remedies for myself!*

— Sharlotte Risley, OTR/L, CHT, licensed occupational therapist and certified hand therapist

Simple, comforting help. An excellent addition to sensible self-help.

— Maggie Letvin, The Beautiful Machine, Inc., fitness expert, teacher, and author of *Maggie's Food Strategy Book, A Guide to Fitness after Fifty*, and *Maggie's Woman's Book*

A very helpful and entertaining book for understanding and treating the many maladies that affect the hands. The author combines medical facts and useful remedies mixed with a great sense of humor.

— Lawrence B. Meyerson, M.D., Chief Physician, The Dermatology and Laser Center,
Irving, Texas, and founder of Clear Reflections Cosmetics

Norma P. Weinberg's Natural Hand Care *provides a much-needed guide for care of the most used and abused member of our body — our hands. It is an encyclopedic treatment of the subject and contains much more information about skin care in general than the title reveals. The author has assembled quite a bit of factual information about hand care in addition to traditional information from our rich herbal heritage and folk wisdom. Anyone with two hands needs to have this book on his book shelf.*

— Nikolaus J. Smeh, M.S., physicist, chemist, and author of
Health Risks in Today's Cosmetics, Creating Your Own Cosmetics — Naturally,
and *Save the Child and Yourself*

Natural Hand Care *is a well-researched, complete, and reliable holistic guide to having attractive, healthy hands. It is filled with easy herbal recipes, colorful anecdotes, and lots of down-to-earth advice. I recommend it!*

— Kathy Keville, director, American Herb Association, and author of
Aromatherapy: The Complete Guide to the Healing Art and *Herbs for Health and Healing*

FOREWORD

Next to the brain, the hand represents humankind's greatest asset. This anatomic marvel has enabled humans to excel over all other species. In reality, the human hand functions to a large degree as an extension of the individual's brain. Witness the truly remarkable capacity of Helen Keller, who was both deaf and blind, to fulfill a meaningful life through her hands.

When humans became bipedal, our hands were relieved of the duty of locomotion and freed to develop into extremely useful and sophisticated instruments. The structures involved in tactile function are highly refined, and the machinery of the hand involves specialized tissues of great delicacy and sophistication. Witness the human thumb, unique in its strength, mobility, and size relative to the digits. With this highly evolved component, our hands have proven successful not only in fundamental tasks of survival but also in drawing, sculpturing, and all of the precise and beautiful things that surround civilization.

Natural Hand Care will appeal to a wide audience of both professional and lay readers. Technical terms are minimized and the thrust of the book is away from the specialized issues of hand anatomy, function, and pathology. Rather, the book explores a wide range of issues related to both how the hand functions as well as the care of its component parts. It is sprinkled with vignettes bringing to the reader historical as well as contemporary issues as diverse as the history of nail polish to the life span of a wart. The book is easy to read, accurate, and — of particular importance — useful.

After reading this text, few if any will ever take their hands for granted. From the perspective of a physician involved in the care of hand problems and traumatic disruptions of the hand, I was enthralled by this text, learned quite a few useful facts, and would recommend it equally to professionals involved in the care of the hand as well as to anyone who takes pride in their hands' appearance and function.

JESSE B. JUPITER, M.D.
Director of Orthopaedic Hand Service, Massachusetts General Hospital
Associate Professor of Orthopaedic Surgery, Harvard Medical School
Editor, *Flynn's Hand Surgery,* 4th edition (Williams & Wilkins, 1990)

CONTENTS

IN SPECIAL GRATITUDE

For the many people who helped make this work possible, including my husband and partner, who served as cheerleader and my power of positive thinking; my friends, for their encouragement, "it-can-be-done" spirit, and assistance beyond the call of duty; and my family, especially my mom, who in her eighth decade remains loving and supportive, and like that famous bunny just keeps going and going and going.

INTUITIVE THINKING

There are easy, natural things we can do to promote our health and the well-being of this planet. It all begins with having the confidence to accept responsibility as caretaker, the capacity to respect each and every voice, and the willingness to try the uncomplicated approach first and, if necessary, advance to the next level of care only as needed. In most cases, the earth has been a nurturing place for its inhabitants, and it seems logical to turn to plants and natural remedies as a first line of defense in helping our bodies deal with temporary malaise.

I attempt to bridge two worlds in this book: the world of Western allopathic medicine, which respects laboratory research and controlled medical studies, and the world of folk herbal medicine, which is tested by a wide range of geographic use and the span of time. These approaches are not antagonistic. Both seek to help the individual to maintain or regain essential health. The allopathic approach often focuses on suppressing overt symptoms of disease (which we typically request in doctor's offices) while the herbalist approach takes the slower route, trying to work with the underlying causes and assist the body in rebuilding natural defenses.

Writing this book has been a fascinating quest. My hope is that you and your family will refer often to this handbook as a commonsense reference on natural care of the hands.

Norma P. Weinberg

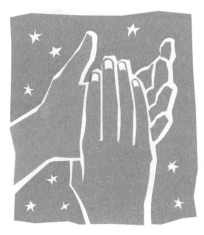

The Undercover Story: Understanding How Your Hands Work

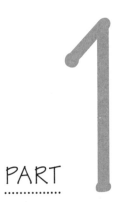

PART 1

CHAPTER 1
A Sense of Touch: Your Communicative and Indispensable Hands

For simplicity, warmth, and sensitivity there is no machine that can equal the human hand.

— Maurice Mességué
C'est la nature qui a' raison

Manus in Latin, *cheir* in Greek, *yad* in Hebrew, *ruka* in Russian, *die Hand* in German — in all languages and in all things, the hand has been significant in man's evolutionary development. The human hand, just four fingers and a countering thumb, is a tool without peer. From the time we awaken until the time we sleep, our indispensable hands help us to fulfill the physical and emotional energies of daily living. Still, we don't give our hands much thought unless they become a problem — unless the skin on our fingertips is cracked and painful, or we break a nail or, even worse, a finger or a wrist. Then we find that expressing ourselves in a discussion, holding hands with a loved one, or even trying to button a shirt becomes a major effort.

Durable and versatile, our hands are our most essential tools. So take some time to understand how they are put together. By understanding how they work and knowing how to care for them naturally, you will ensure yourself a lifetime of healthy, strong, and limber hands.

FLEXIBILITY: MOVING AND USING YOUR FINGERS AND HANDS

Our hands give us the capability to reach out and act on our world. Think about how many different ways you call on your fingers to help you every day. Spend a moment and try this exercise:

◆ Pick up a pencil.
◆ Hold a key.
◆ Open a door.
◆ Clasp a coffee mug.

If you study the back of the hand, you will notice interesting distinctions about the movement abilities of each of the fingers. We can stretch our fingers far apart as well as touch the thumb to each of the fingers. But individually, each finger has its own particular characteristics that add to or limit the flexibility of the hand.

The *middle finger*, also the longest finger, is the most limited in motion by its attachment to the five metacarpal bones between the wrist and the fingers.

The *index finger*, or *forefinger*, is usually the second longest finger on the hand. It has the greatest range of independent movement. Because of this flexibility, we use the index finger for pointing and for beckoning.

The *ring finger* does not bend or straighten without being accompanied, at least partially, by one or both of the fingers on either side. This is partly because its tendons are connected on either side by a band of fibers. Because this finger is protected in movement by fingers on either side, it became the choice for ring wearing.

The *little finger*, or *pinkie*, cannot bend or flex on its own. This circumstance is a protection for its position, size, and susceptibility to hard knocks. (The word "pinkie" comes from the Dutch word *pinkje*, which means "little finger.")

The *thumb* has a range of varied movements. Its position on the hand, in opposition to the other fingers, allows it to grasp and pick up objects. Except for some primates, no other known animals have this capability. This flexibility of action is what allows us a strong, firm grip and the dexterity and precision to hold an object in any position, to touch it from all sides, and to release it. Without this unique thumb, we would be able only to roll the object within our hand.

Dexterity

Notice how the hand is capable of delicate work, such as picking up individual grains of rice or fine pins from a carpet. That same hand can also squeeze a rubber ball or hang on to a heavy box. Biomechanical engineers have tried for centuries to duplicate the remarkable human hand, but with only limited success.

Just think about the distinct holds and the different finger grips that a baseball pitcher uses in throwing a fastball, a curveball, a knuckleball, and a slider. Notice the contrasting ways you grasp a screwdriver, a wrench, and a file. Human hands are capable of so many patterns of grips. We call on these precision holds every single day:

- *tip grip* (to thread a needle)
- *lateral grip* (to hold a key)
- *palm grip* (to grab a hammer or paintbrush)
- *hook grip* (to carry a suitcase or hangers)

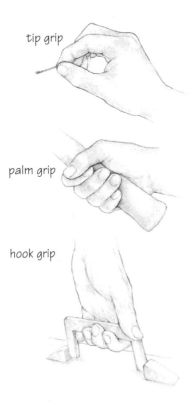

tip grip

lateral grip

palm grip

hook grip

The gorilla's hands, with their tapering fingers, appear very similar to our human hands. However, a distinctly different combination of muscles in the palm, thumb, and fingers restricts the ability of these parts to function separately from one another. The ape's grip is strong, but its hold is a power grip, not the human precision grip.

In 1959, after a decade of excavations, British anthropologists Mary and Louis Leakey announced the important discovery of fossil finds of early man in the Olduvai Gorge, in the East African Rift Valley of Tanzania. This valley, dry for most of the year, yielded evidence of a specimen of early man who lived about 1.75 million years ago named *Homo habilis* (or "handy" man). The fossil hand bones of *Homo habilis* revealed skeletal capacity to use the precision grip thought necessary to make primitive tools such as axes, choppers, cleavers, and spearheads, and indeed remains of stone tools were found nearby. This was the earliest find documenting human capability for precision grip.

Unintentional Sign Language: Talking with Your Hands

Through our hand movements, we tell others a great deal about ourselves without always being aware of our messages. Here are some examples of hand signs to be aware of when seated in a group around a table:

Hand Language	Implied Meaning
Hands and fingers out front, plainly in view on the table	I have nothing to hide.
Arms folded over chest	A bit defensive; challenging; I'm not convinced.
Chin resting on one fist	I'm listening, but I'm not sure yet.
Both hands resting on a table, side-by-side, palms-down, fingers flat	Okay, I agree with what you are saying.
Leaning forward, chin resting on both fists	I'm interested.
Leaning back, both hands resting on the lap or fingers busy with a pen, pencil, or paperclip	I'm somewhere else.

Communicating With Your Fists

According to Walter Sorrell, author of *The Story of the Human Hand,* it's possible to identify an individual's personality traits by observing that person's fist and the position of the thumb in relation to the fingers. If you want clues to someone's basic nature, inspect the way he or she makes a fist and compare it with this list. Good luck!

- A thumb hidden inside a fist is what we see in a newborn infant. An adult who hides the thumb in the shell of the fingers shows tension or restrained emotion, a desire for protection, and a dependence on other people.
- A thumb that covers clenched fingers is the sign of a high-strung individual, an ever-ready fighter, a person who surrenders easily to emotions.
- A thumb resting alongside a fist is indicative of counterbalance and a sense of reason dominating emotion; this may be the posture of a strong-willed yet successful person who is able to abide by a spirit of restraint.
- A thumb resting under the index finger but peeking through the fist tells us this person is shy, reserved, a bit suspicious, and somewhat anxious.
- A thumb that stretches far out from the palm forming a right angle with the index finger — the classic hitchhiker's pose — is indicative of self-confidence, strength, and the capacity to direct other people, singly or in groups.

A SENSE OF TOUCH

The average adult handshake exerts 90 pounds of force and can be as much as 150 pounds of force.

Have you ever noticed how dogs will "sing" at the sound of a violin? They are hearing vibrations that we can't hear. Or perhaps you have seen a bear (from a suitable distance) following a scented trail to some sweet honey or berries that our sense of smell is not able to detect. Maybe you've observed a hawk hovering high in the air and then, sensing minute motion, swooping down to catch the tiniest of prey.

HANDISMS

- Crossing your fingers to wish someone good luck goes far back to a belief in magic that can tie things together.

- Clapping hands was a traditional way to call the spirits. Today, it is most often done to express applause. Or can it be a way of thanking the spirits for helping the performer do well?

- Handshakes did not always represent the mutual courtesy they do today. One of the oldest gestures in the world, handshaking has symbolized throughout history a pledge of good faith — and proof of the lack of a weapon. You would shake someone's right hand on meeting and on parting to make certain your acquaintance wasn't holding a dagger. (In my opinion, handshaking is a custom we could replace today with a hug — it would save a great deal of hand-washing and germ-spreading.)

- The thumbs-down gesture is a centuries-old expression of rejection, disapproval, or condemnation. Its opposite, thumbs-up, is a newer gesture signifying encouragement or approval.

And if you have lived with a pet feline, you are most likely in awe of the taste buds of this creature who favors some foods and disdains or avoids others.

We do not hear, smell, see, or taste with the same acuity as other animals. But we are at the head of the pack in the development of our sense of touch — especially in our keenly responsive fingertips and hands. Human fingertips harbor an incredible repository of sensory nerves — approximately one hundred nerve endings per square centimeter. In contrast, less sensitive body parts have only about five sensory nerves per square centimeter.

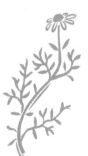

Each fingertip is imprinted with an individualized print pattern. Using fingerprints as a unique means of establishing human identity dates back centuries, at least, to the time when venerable Chinese merchants used their thumbprints as legal seals of identity. But fingerprints exist for more reasons than to serve as a means of identification. Our corrugated, slightly rough fingertips and palms also serve to improve our grasp and enhance our perceptions of touch and pressure.

Fingerprints for Touch

Fingerprints are patterns of fine ridges, separated by grooves or furrows, on the epidermal skin of the palm-side of the fingers and hands. This imprinted part of our skin is perfectly adapted for touch, with no hairs or sebaceous (oil) glands to impede contact with a surface. Instead, these fine ridges are dotted with rows of abundant sweat glands, up to eighteen sweat pores per millimeter. The perspiration supplied by these sweat glands helps to lubricate the skin, keeping the fingertips supple and enhancing our ability to both touch and grasp. As we touch objects with our hands, the rough ridges of our fingerprints, along with our sensory nerves (which are embedded in the furrows), create a friction between our hand and the object that enhances our ability to feel the object's texture, temperature, and solidity. If our fingertip skin were finely polished on the surface, we would have a greatly reduced capacity for tactile sense.

Fingerprints for Identification

Fingerprints were first documented by pattern types in 1823 by Dr. Jan Purkinje, a professor of physiology at the University of Breslau. He was the father of the science of fingerprinting for individual identification. Particularly useful for verifying the identity of criminals, fingerprinting asked only to match shapes of the ridge patterns and their positions on the ten fingers in order to prove that a set of prints belonged to a particular individual. By June of 1897, Sir William James Herschel, a British official serving in Bengal, India, was able to begin a fingerprint system throughout the subcontinent. In 1901, the Bertillon system in England and Wales had identified 462 criminals. In 1904, the number grew to 5,155, and by 1905, there were fingerprint records of eighty thousand people. Today, the FBI has more than 200 million fingerprints on file and is able to identify the prints of about forty thousand criminal suspects annually.

Although no two sets of fingerprints are alike, there are several general patterns. The ridges on the fingertips may form arches, loops, or whorls. Loops are the most frequent, accounting for about 60 percent of all patterns. People of Asian descent seem to display a higher percentage of whorl patterns. Men's ridges are usually thicker than women's. Women tend to have more arches and fewer whorl patterns than men, although it has not been entirely possible to determine a person's gender or race by his or her fingerprints.

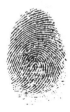 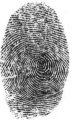 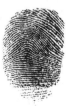

loop   whorl   arch

Noseprints are thought to be as reliable an index of identity for dogs as are fingerprints for humans.

Relying on Touch

It's not often that we focus on the genius of the design, but the human hand has the capacity to feel and act simultaneously. Our hands are our tactile eyes. We gather data through the sense of touch in our fingertips and palms, and use these details for problem solving and to frame the way we perceive our surroundings.

Helen Keller was able to "listen" to music by placing her hand on the radio and feeling the rhythm and vibrations of the various instruments. And what of the hand that produced the music? What makes a Jascha Heifetz, a Beethoven, a Pablo Casals? We still do not know how much the brain learns from the sensitive touch of the fingers in order to aid the hand in producing the symphony.

Louis Braille used the sense of touch to make the hands see for the blind. Born in France, he lost his sight in an accident at the age of three. Educated with sighted children at the village school, he realized that the visually impaired needed books to learn. By the age of 15, he was already working on a system of dot-writing for instantaneous fingertip identification of letters and numbers. A French army officer, Charles Barbier, had already worked out a system of communicating at night on the battlefield with embossed dots and dashes. He shared this idea with Braille, who simplified it to using six raised points or dots in sixty-three combinations for printing, writing, and musical notations. Louis Braille died two years before his system was officially adopted in the schools.

Question: Which body parts are the most sensitive to touch?

Answer: They're probably not what you think — our most sensitive touch receptors are the tongue and the fingertips.

Hands On: Touch Aptitude

Ralph, a friend of mine, was born blind and has only his hands with which to "see" his environment. He suggested this sensitivity session. I hope it will bring home the talent in your fingertips.

The next time you have the luxury of leisurely shopping for groceries, spend a few extra moments at the fruit and vegetable bins with your eyes closed. You'll find that your sense of touch provides you with much information.

Texture. Close your eyes and let your hand tell you about the silky texture of a tomato, or the similarities in the bumpy grains of lemons, oranges, or avocados.

Shape. Notice how you know the shape of an onion, in contrast to a bulb of garlic. Feel how the hand can discriminate an apple from a pear, a banana from grapes.

Contrast. When you reach the checkout counter and put your hand in your pocket, notice how your hand informs you that the fabric lining the inside pocket, maybe a cotton, is different from the outside of the jacket, perhaps a wool.

Size. Then feel the various sizes and smooth or rough edges of the coins in your pocket change. Most likely you can identify the coins without having to look.

Feel. If you are paying with a plastic credit card, notice, when you sign the receipt, how you instinctively know the tactile sensation of holding a pencil versus a pen.

TOUCH YOUR FINGER, TOUCH YOUR NOSE

Can you do it? How attuned are you to the bounds of your body? Here's a basic test of coordination and spatial awareness. Close your eyes (but not until you read the rest of the instructions!). Spread your arms out at your sides like an eagle's wings. With your index fingers leading, bring your hands together until the fingers of both hands meet tip-to-tip. Then, in turn, touch your nose with each index finger. It may take a few tries to complete this task successfully. Between each try, open your eyes and take a few steps to reset.

An Everyday Warm-Up Stretch and Massage for Your Hands

We work our hands hard and rarely take the time to care properly for them. Here are some basic limbering exercises and easy massages to do each morning while you are still in bed. They will tone and stretch your hand and arm muscles, stimulate circulation, and limber up your joints for the day ahead.

Step 1: Stretch. Reach your arms over your head and stretch your whole body. Feel your spine elongate. Relax. Now, reach your arms out to the sides. Stretch your rib cage and breathe deeply in and out. Notice how your abdomen rises on the inhale and falls on the exhale.

Step 2: Backs-of-hands massage. Rub the palm of the left hand over the back of the right hand; repeat the action with the palm of the right hand rubbing the back of the left hand, as if washing the hands. This stimulates circulation and warms the hands.

Step 3: Finger milking. With your right hand, "milk" each finger and thumb on the left hand (as if you were milking a cow or a goat). Begin closer to your knuckles and gently but firmly pull, squeeze, and work your way down to the fingertips. Repeat on the opposite hand.

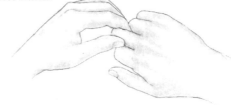

Step 4: Nail press. With the thumb and index finger of the opposite hand, press on each nail and do a gentle twist and rock, to bring circulation to the fingertips.

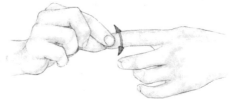

Step 5: Wrist circles. While lying on your back, form large, lazy circles with your arms, using your shoulders. Gradually work down to smaller and smaller circles until you are making just small, graceful circles with your wrists.

Step 6: Shake it out. It's time to sit up on the edge of the bed. With your arms hanging down by your sides, shake out both hands — first, loosely as a scarecrow, and then, rotating the thumb toward you and then away from you in a motion similar to the central post of a washing machine.

Step 7: Fists. Keeping your arms down, open and close your fists and squeeze your fingers into your palm (watch out for long nails!). This applies some pressure and encourages circulation.

Your hands are now ready to meet the day!

THE POWER OF PHYSICAL TOUCH

Touch is perhaps our first sense to develop and the last to take its leave. For newborns, contact is automatic. Even before the eyes open, a baby's hands reach out for comfort and warmth.

Our hands not only feed us information about our surroundings but also enhance our emotional contact with others and the world around us. Sometimes we are not even aware that we are receiving this sustenance. Touch is an integral part of our sensory system, but at no time does it affect us more than when it is a human touch. Whether we are giving or receiving the contact, it affects not only how we react but also with whom and what. The human touch can make you roll with laughter, lull you to sleep, or break through emotional barriers and elicit tears of sorrow or loneliness. No other human sense can arouse us as touch can. Hearing, vision, and smell are all secondary.

Yet we tend to take touch as much for granted as we do breathing, until it becomes absent from or infrequent in our lives. As humans, we need to touch and to be touched. The connection between touch and well-being is far more than skin deep. The amount of physical contact in our lives plays a vital role in our mental and physical health and in our development.

There is a direct connection between our tactile sense and the nervous system and brain. We find that our inner emotions and psychological states can be deeply affected by whom or what we touch. It's almost as if we have an innate compulsion to touch. Our eyes perceive the object in space, but we understand more about its three-dimensionality by contacting the surface. Museums are very aware of our need to handle objects — just notice the "PLEASE DON'T TOUCH" signs in every sculpture gallery.

It was a custom in ancient Greece — continued by some even today — to carry a small, smooth stone such as amber or jade in one's pocket as a "fingering piece" or "worry bead." Fingers on a cool, hard surface offer a sense of quiet.

A Touching Story

I travel a great deal to share my thoughts on how to stay healthy naturally. A favorite talk is "Herbs for Romance." Recently, I was fortunate to be speaking on a round-the-world cruise to a mature crowd. I was not sure who would be present for this subject matter. However, at the appointed time, the room was full.

I began by sharing the information about how more romance occurs between the ears than below the waist (a maxim of Dr. Ruth Westheimer). It is important to set aside time for love, I told my audience, and spoke of utilizing all of the senses to create a mood.

Touch is one of the senses that, to my mind, plays a major role in romance. Touch connotes responsiveness and care. A skillful caress can make the body sing, while the play of love may begin with the language of holding hands. I gently suggested that a first step might be to give one's special partner at least three hugs a day.

Touching is just as therapeutic as being touched; the healer, the giver of touch, is simultaneously healed . . . . Even touch so subtle as to be overlooked doesn't go unnoticed by the unconscious mind.

— Diane Ackerman
The Natural History of the Senses

One gentleman came to speak to me afterward. He said that he did not have a partner because his wife of fifty years had passed on. Not wanting to disappoint him on this long journey, I told him that I would be willing to give him a hug whenever he needed one. That was the beginning of much fun aboard ship, and possibly a new friend for life. And all it took was a little hug.

My "Fanny" Club, or Touch Power

This is another cruise story. After one of my talks aboard the ship, two very proper British ladies approached and asked if I had any natural remedies to suggest for lower back pain. They had been to sick bay, they said, and the doctor had given them a form of aspirin, but they needed something more. I told them that I had some St.-John's-wort oil, which reduces pain and is an anti-inflammatory herb, in my tote. I would be willing to share some as long as they had no allergies or sensitivities. They admitted to none so I suggested we visit the ladies' room together.

I set my bag down on the powder room counter and proceeded to search for the elusive oil. When I turned around, both of these dignified women had dropped their drawers. With a smile, I asked if it might not have been a better idea for each of them to tell me their names before getting so comfortable.

In a few moments, I had rubbed each of their lower backs with the oil and they were very pleased. It was the "hands-on" healing experience they wanted. Within hours, the word had spread, and the beginnings of my "fanny" club were underway. Everywhere I went on that ship, people followed my fanny, seeking a healing, hands-on remedy. The power of touch cannot be underrated!

> A healing relationship can be a loving touch, a positive expectancy, the sense of self-worth, even a bit of magic. Healers in all traditions hold the power to evoke this golden thread of healing.
>
> — Excerpted from "The Healing Relationship," by Jerry Solfvin, in *Healers on Healing*, edited by Richard Carlson and Benjamin Shield

AYURVEDIC GEM THERAPY

Ayurvedic gem therapy is a healing practice that relies on energy being directed to the hands and then to the body through the power of touch. If you love wearing jewels on your fingers, this is definitely a pleasing way to affect your psyche and perhaps your inner health. You will have to decide for yourself what you think of its therapeutic value. Here's how gem therapy works.

Ayurveda, a healing system focused on the well-being of body, mind, and spirit, is based on the ancient Vedic texts of

India dating from about 2500 B.C.E. The term comes from two Indian words: *ayur,* or "life," and *veda,* "knowledge." Within the practice of Ayurveda there are various therapies aligned with Hindu astrology to treat physical, mental, and spiritual disorders. Gemstone therapy is one such treatment and has been used for thousands of years in India for preventive, therapeutic, and remedial purposes.

Gemstones are mythically connected to the planets in our solar system. It is believed that the planets exert an influence on all aspects of human life. In addition, the way the gems are formed inextricably ties them to earth elements. When worn, gems are said to align the individual with the healing forces of nature. Particular precious stones are selected for rings based on their influences on earth elements and to act as a medium for the transmission of energy from the planet to the wearer.

Finger rings made for Ayurvedic gem therapy are set so that the gemstones come into direct contact with the skin. By wearing the jewels on specific fingers and hands, a person is strengthened or defended by this amulet. The chart below will show you the desired finger, the gem, the influencing planet, and the earth element.

The Ayurvedic healing properties attributed to each precious stone are described on the next page. When you wear the gems for therapeutic purposes, the stones should be of significant size — if possible, at least two carats. Less expensive substitutes are offered, but these are not felt to be as powerful as the "real" thing.

THE TOUCH OF GEMS

Finger	Gem	Ruled by Planet	Ruled by Element
Little finger	emerald	Mars, Mercury	earth
Ring finger	diamond, ruby, pearl	Sun or Moon, Venus	water
Middle finger	blue sapphire	Saturn	air
Index finger	yellow sapphire	Jupiter, Saturn	ether

Emerald. The green emerald promotes healing, energizes and strengthens the breath, and increases flexibility and adaptability of the mind. It should be set in silver or gold and worn on the little finger. Possible substitutes are green tourmaline or green zircon.

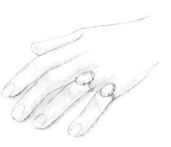

Ruby. The red ruby — the gem of kings — strengthens the will, gives insight, promotes independence, and enhances power. Rubies are usually set in gold and worn on the ring finger of the right hand. A possible substitute is garnet.

Pearl and diamond. The white pearl and diamond are symbols of purity and light. These gems calm the emotions, nourish the nerves and body tissues, and strengthen the female reproductive system. Pearls and diamonds are usually set in silver and worn on the ring finger of the left hand. Possible substitutes are clear quartz crystal or moonstone.

Blue sapphire. The blue sapphire strengthens bones, increases longevity, and helps calm nerves and emotions. It has the power to ward off negative energies while promoting tranquillity and concentration. It should be set in either gold or silver and worn on the middle finger. A possible substitute is amethyst.

Yellow sapphire. The yellow sapphire is considered the best stone for generally promoting health and fostering recuperation. It is usually set in gold and worn on the index finger. Possible substitutes are yellow topaz or citrine.

If gem therapy is of interest to you, save this information in a wish list to show to someone before your birthday or anniversary! You may also find it helpful to read some of the many books available or visit some of the web sites on the Internet devoted to Ayurveda, or visit a physician skilled in Ayurveda.

CHAPTER 2
The Hand Bone's Connected to the . . .

*White or black, brown or yellow, small or large, marked with
the ridges and wrinkles of old age or youthful . . . and
untouched, they are the masterpiece which no artist has
equaled, no inventor has ever duplicated.*
— Paul Tabori, *The Book of the Hand*

If two characteristics could describe the dexterity of our hands,
they would be the skill in bringing the tips of our thumbs and
fingers together and the exquisite sensitivity in our fingertips.
Now, let's take a closer look at the undercover network systems
of the hand that make movement and sensitivity possible: the
skin, bones, muscles, nerves, and vascular functions.

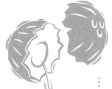

HAND SURFACES:
THEY'RE NOT JUST A PROTECTIVE SHIELD!

The skin that covers our hands fulfills many obligations. It
functions as a protective shield and, just as importantly, is the
locus for our sense of touch. With rich nerve endings, the skin
responds to a myriad of sensations and at times seems to be the
"eyes" of the hand. Discreetly placed oil glands secrete sebum
(a fatty, oily substance) to moisturize and waterproof our skin,
and sweat glands excrete toxins to regulate body heat. The skin
also produces vitamin D in the presence of sunlight and partici-
pates in cutaneous respiration (the absorption of oxygen and
the giving off of watery substances).

Our skin is our first line of defense against the outside
world. It heats and cools us, warns other body systems of
invaders, and retains and excretes our bodily fluids. It's a truly
amazing, waterproof, washable, and flexible substance that is
able to self-mend and self-renew.

The Many Layers of Skin

So many of our experiences are transmitted through the skin. Ultrasensitive receptors allow us to perceive touch, pressure, cold, warmth, and pain, and combinations of these same sensory modalities expand our perceptions to include wondrous feelings like tickle, wetness, softness, and hardness as well as surface texture, form, force, and weight.

To get a better picture of the structure and function of the skin, let's meander through some of its many faces.

The stratum corneum, the outermost layer of the epidermis, is made up of flat, toughened cells. It is about 20 cell layers deep, averaging only about .0004 inches (or $1/100$ mm) in thickness. This outermost layer is the last stage in the life cycle of a skin cell, just before it is shed. We lose thousands of dead skin cells from the stratum corneum every time we scratch, rub, or wash our hands.

The tough cells in this horny layer keep our bodily fluids in and environmental fluids out, as well as protect the delicate, living cells beneath from injury, dryness, and attacks by bacteria and harmful chemicals. A thin coating of sebum helps keep this outermost layer of skin soft, pliable, and waterproof.

Skin abrasions and exposure to detergents and solvents can weaken the barrier properties of the stratum corneum and make it feel rough to the touch. When the skin is damaged by frequent pressure or friction, this outer layer can clump together in corns (bumps) and calluses (thickened skin). Fortunately, the protective surface of the outer skin can be restored by topical treatment with natural creams and salves (see chapter 7).

AMING SKIN

If I asked you to name all the organs of the body, I bet that the skin would not even make your list. Yet this continuous, resilient outer covering that encases our being is our largest organ. The skin, which weighs between 5 and 10 pounds (2.3 to 4.5 kg), is also the body's heaviest organ.

The epidermis is the self-repairing, self-renewing layer of the skin that includes and lies just below the stratum corneum. It averages .005 inches (or 0.07 mm) in thickness and is made up of scalelike cells composed of a waxy, water-proof protein called keratin. These skin cells live for 15 to 30 days before being flattened and pushed upward by new cells produced from below. The epidermal skin on the palms of the hands and soles of the feet is normally thicker than anywhere else on the body.

The epidermis is also the first line of defense for the body's immune system. With a pH around 5.0, the epidermis shows an acid mantle to microorganisms that deters their invasion of the skin. Too-frequent washing and the use of antibiotics may upset this natural balance and lead to infection. The epidermis is also seeded with *Langerhans cells,* which are alert to foreign substances and signal the body's immune system to kick into action.

The lowest layers of the epidermis are where the skin pigment, called *melanin,* is formed. *Melanocyte* cells manufacture the melanin that produces the intensity of our particular skin and hair color according to genetic DNA recipes. Differences in skin color are due only to the amount, type, and arrangement of the melanin within the epidermis — skin color is otherwise the same for all humans through most of the other layers of the skin.

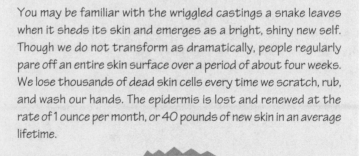

You may be familiar with the wriggled castings a snake leaves when it sheds its skin and emerges as a bright, shiny new self. Though we do not transform as dramatically, people regularly pare off an entire skin surface over a period of about four weeks. We lose thousands of dead skin cells every time we scratch, rub, and wash our hands. The epidermis is lost and renewed at the rate of 1 ounce per month, or 40 pounds of new skin in an average lifetime.

The protective purpose of melanin is to absorb ultraviolet rays from the sun, thereby protecting us from sun damage to our skin. The darker the natural color of the skin, the more melanin is present, and the better adapted the body is to life under the sun.

The dermis, or true skin, is a spongy, connective tissue whose major components include collagen (for structure) and elastin (for elasticity) proteins. It averages .078 inches (or 1 to 2 mm) in thickness. The dermis houses the hair follicles, which function as ultrasensitive touch receptors. It is directly connected to the nervous system, the glands that produce sebum and sweat, lymph vessels, and 25 percent of the body's blood supply.

Keratin, a major component of our skin cells, is a product of the food we eat. Our body breaks food down into amino acids, the building blocks of protein. In the skin, protein globules link up in chemical chains called protofibrils. These chains wind together to form microfibrils, and the rope-like microfibrils are woven into keratin. Every hoof, horn, claw, nail, bill, beak, feather, fur, and hair, as far as we know, is made of a pattern of woven keratin.

Examining Your Hands

Look at your hands, front and back. You've probably noticed that the surface texture of the skin changes according to age, health, climate, and the environment. But if you observe closely, you will notice a subtle difference between the skin on the back of the hand and that on the palm, no matter what the circumstance.

The back of the hand. The skin on the back of the hand, called the *dorsal skin,* is thin and pliable. It is easily separated or pinched away from underlying tissues. This suppleness is essential for the movement and flexibility of the fingers.

The palm. The skin on the palm of the hand, called the *volar skin,* is thick and hairless, rich in sensory receptors, and supplied with sweat glands that help to lower the body's temperature and eliminate toxins. This skin is firmly attached, not as easily separated as is the skin on the back of the hand. Its design allows us to grasp and hold objects (see "Fingerprints for Touch" on page 8).

Hair. Notice the fine, soft hairs on the back of the hand (fair-haired folks may need a magnifying glass). There are about 120 hairs per square inch on the hands, or about 15 to 20 hairs per square centimeter. These hairs have an important role as protective warning devices. When bent, hair follicles on the skin's surface activate sensitive touch receptors.

Downy hairs on the backs of the fingers and hands usually grow only a fraction of an inch. If you look carefully, on a sunny day, you will notice small patches of hair on the fingers, and might be surprised to see that this hair is growing only in one direction — angled toward the pinkie side of the hand. It's not often that we spend this much time on tiny details, but it's interesting getting to know our bodies a bit better.

Fingernails. Fingernails protect the upper surface of the fingertips and help us to grasp, scratch, and pinch. Nails also provide a form of external stability for the softer skin around the fingertip. (See part 2, beginning on page 47, for everything you ever wanted to know about taking care of your nails.)

Lines and creases. Looking at the palm surface of your hands, see that the skin on both your fingers and palms is impregnated with lines or creases. Believe it or not, these lines and creases each play a different role. (I am not talking about palm reading here.) Cup your palm and you will notice *flex folds* located where the skin is connected to deeper tissues. These lines permit the hand to close without the skin folding over or bunching. As an example of what it might be like not to have lines and creases here, think of when you have wrapped a package and the paper bunched up before you could secure it with ribbon or string!

LET ME READ YOUR PALM!

For centuries, the hand has been thought of as a symbolic link to the psyche and the soul. Palmistry, a mystical profession, attempts to analyze a person's character or predict his or her destiny by studying the features of the hand, especially the palm. With roots in ancient Egypt, Greece, and China, the Gypsies were the group who brought palmistry to Europe from Asia during the Renaissance.

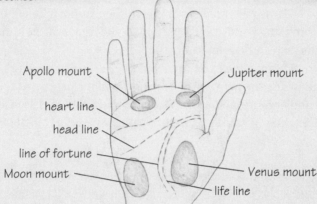

Apollo mount — Jupiter mount
heart line
head line
line of fortune
Moon mount — Venus mount
life line

Here's a brief overview of the important features. Hand reading involves studying the length and depth of the four principal lines in the palm: the head line, the heart line, the life line, and the line of fortune. The *heart line* relates to affection. The *line of fortune or fate* is a predictor of success or failure in life. The nature of the *head line* allies with a person's intelligence, and the length and constancy of the *life line* connects to longevity or bouts with illness.

There are also seven mounts, or small rises, on the palm (some of which are shown above). Each mount takes its name either from a heavenly body or a mythological being. Beginning with the mount on the index finger, they are Jupiter, Saturn, Apollo, Mercury, Mars, Moon, and Venus. The development or lack of fullness of each mount is said to reveal features of character. Jupiter represents ambition; Saturn is wisdom and luck. Apollo is intelligence; Mercury is the ability to communicate; Mars is bravery; Luna, or the moon, is linked to the imagination or intuition; and Venus represents vitality and sensuality.

Because fortunetelling provides many opportunities for fraud, the practice is against the law in much of the United States and in some western countries, although you may find palm readers at summer Renaissance fairs.

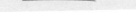

Bones of the Hand

Anatomically, the bones of the hand can be divided into three parts: those in the fingers, the palm, and the wrist.

The *fingers*, or *phalanges*, are formed by fourteen phalangeal bones. There are three of these bones in each finger, but only two in the thumb.

The *palm*, or *metacarpus*, the main part of the hand, has five metacarpal bones.

The *wrist*, or *carpus*, has eight bones that connect the forearm to the hand. Tendons connect the bones of the hands with the bones of the lower arm.

This complex and yet adaptable skeletal framework is what allows us the range of fine and gross movements in our fingers, hands, wrists, and arms. The hand can adapt and adjust to perform massive tasks as well as delicate, precise functions.

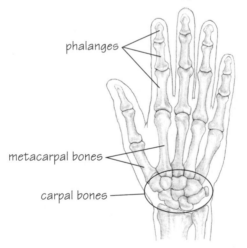

phalanges

metacarpal bones

carpal bones

Joints and Spaces in the Hands

A joint is a junction between the ends of two or more bones in the skeleton. A synovial joint is surrounded by the joint capsule, a layer of fibrous tissue with an inner lining called the synovial membrane. This membrane produces a protective, transparent fluid that lubricates and nourishes the joint surfaces. The various types of joints in our fingers, hands, and wrists permit us to bend, flex, and rotate our fingers, wrists, and elbows. (For more information, see chapter 9, beginning on page 164.)

Muscles, Tendons, and Ligaments of the Hand

The muscles of the hand rarely act alone; rather, they function as part of an interactive group. All normal movements are a balance between the opposing forces of each of the muscles. There are twenty small muscle groups for independent finger movements, plus an additional fourteen muscle groups in the forearm.

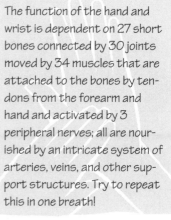

The function of the hand and wrist is dependent on 27 short bones connected by 30 joints moved by 34 muscles that are attached to the bones by tendons from the forearm and hand and activated by 3 peripheral nerves; all are nourished by an intricate system of arteries, veins, and other support structures. Try to repeat this in one breath!

Thumb muscles and movements. There are nine muscles that contribute to the flexibility and strength of the thumb. These muscles allow the thumb greater mobility and range of motion than that of the other fingers because the thumb requires more strength in order to oppose the pressure exerted by four fingers.

If you've ever crushed a Ping-Pong ball or a soft drink can in the palm of your hand, you know it's a relatively easy task because the thumb plays a major role. But try cracking a fresh egg lying across your palm, grasped evenly by the four fingers, with no help from the thumb. (This is tougher than it sounds.)

Connective tissue. Connective tissue provides the support for numerous structures in the body. In the hands, connective tissue exists as bundles of collagen and elastin. These bundles of ribbonlike protein fibers have three major functions: to separate or connect structures; to cushion and protect; and to maintain the shape of the hands, palms, and fingers.

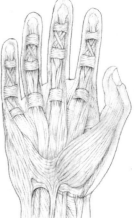

Every muscle, tendon, ligament, nerve, and blood vessel is surrounded by connective tissue that separates or connects these structures.

Tendons. Tendons connect muscles to bones. All of the muscle groups in the hand are joined to bones by more than twenty long tendons. These tendons enter the hand by passing under a large "wristband" tendon in the wrist, and then go forward to form a crisscross pattern around each finger. Think of muscles and tendons as the under-skin — a support web — for the bones of the hand.

Ligaments. Ligaments are dense fibrous bands that provide stability and connect bones. They act as connection points, coordination and guidance units, and restraint mechanisms.

Nerves of the Hand

Three major nerves in the hand allow us to feel sensation, experience motion, and participate in fine, delicate movements.

The *median nerve* is the chief nerve for precision grip. This nerve controls finger flexion (bending fingers in to the palm) and wrist flexion (bending the wrist down) as well as sensation in the palm-side surfaces of the thumb, index, middle, and half of the ring finger. It is the median nerve that innervates (supplies a stimulus to) the muscles that control thumb opposition. It passes through the carpal tunnel.

The *radial nerve* supplies sensation to the back of the hand. It affects the muscles that extend the arm, forearm, hand, and fingers.

The *ulnar nerve* is another motor nerve of the muscles of the hand. It works with the median nerve to innervate the muscles responsible for fine movements of the hand, such as playing the guitar, writing, sewing, or typing.

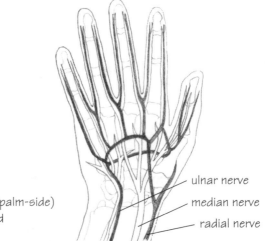

front (palm-side)
of hand

ulnar nerve

median nerve

radial nerve

The Hand's Circulatory System

Nutrients and oxygen are carried to the tissues of the hand through the arteries, capillaries, and veins that direct the bloodstream. The nutrient- and oxygen-rich blood coming from the heart passes first through the *brachial artery* of the upper arm and then through either the *radial* or *ulnar artery* (vessels on the right and left sides of the forearm, respectively). Any blockage in the radial or ulnar artery affects circulation and may cause swelling and pain in the hand and a sensitivity to cold. A blockage in an artery may also cause a bluish, mottled, or pale discoloration of the hand.

36–24–36

This is a wonderful story that tells how the ancient Greek sculptors determined the proportions for the ideal human body.

Polyclitus, a sculptor from Sicyon, drew up the first guidelines for body sculpture dimensions using the human hand as his basic measuring unit. His guidelines were followed for centuries. Here's some of what he recommended for sculpting the perfect figure:

◆ Eighteen thumbs would represent the height of the model body.

◆ The nose, the longest toe, and the thumb were to be equal in length.

◆ The foot, the face, and the hand were also to be equal in length.

◆ The neck was to be twice as thick as the wrist.

◆ The circumference of the wrist was to be twice that of the thumb.

◆ The thumb was to be one-third the length of the hand.

◆ The circumference of the fist was to be equal to the length of the foot.

◆ The length of the index finger determined the width of the hand and the foot.

HANDEDNESS

Handedness is the tendency to use one hand more than the other for skilled actions. About 90 percent of all adults are right-handed. Each side claims their own talents. Lefties (I'm one) have more hurdles to cross in this culture, as most tools and biomechanical designs are engineered for right-handers. (For information on left-handed tools, props, and associations, see page 252 in "Resources.") Here are some statistics for those who relish numbers:

- About one person in every ten is left-handed.
- It is in the seventh month of life that a baby begins to favor one hand over the other; until then, all babies are ambidextrous.
- There are at least twenty million lefties in the United States. Worldwide there are about five hundred million lefties.
- Only about two in one hundred people are ambidextrous.
- There are more than twice as many left-handed men as women.
- The toilet handle is "lefty-friendly."

FAMOUS LEFTIES

Alexander the Great, Michelangelo, Leonardo daVinci, Beethoven, Pablo Picasso, F. Lee Bailey, Harry Truman, Gerald Ford, Ringo Starr, Paul McCartney, Judy Garland, Charlie Chaplin, Kim Novak, Robert Redford, Marilyn Monroe, Babe Ruth, Billy the Kid, Whoopi Goldberg, Jerry Seinfeld, Fran Drescher, Jay Leno, Jimmy Connors.

Most likely, you've always considered yourself either a "lefty" or a "righty," and indeed, most people are predominately one-handed. Perhaps, though, you are ambidextrous and write with your right hand and bowl with your left hand. Try a few of these hand and thumb dominance tests to determine your true strengths.

◆ Clasp your hands. Which thumb is on top? Are you right- or left-thumb dominant? (If your left thumb covers the right thumb, some psychologists would say that instinctive feelings, emotion, and intuition act as driving forces in your life. Right thumb covering left? You are realistic, a rational thinker, and base your decisions on reasoning.)

◆ Look at your thumbnails. The thumbnail on the side of your preferred hand is usually broader. You may notice a difference in the size of the moons on each thumb, too.

◆ When you clap or rub your hands, your preferred hand hits the other, which plays the more passive role.

◆ Draw a profile of a face, including an eye, the nose, and lips. When lefties draw a profile, they almost always have the person facing to the right. Right-handers face the profile to the left.

If you are a lefty, substitute a #2 H pencil for the #2. It has a much tougher lead that hardly smears.

CHAPTER 3
Hand to Mouth: Nutrition for the Nails, Skin, Bones, and Joints

Grasshoppers are said to live on air because, I suppose,
their singing makes their lack of food a light matter.
— Philo, *Contemplative Life* 4

What can your hands and fingernails tell you about your overall health? A keen observer will detect many clues. The color and temperature of fingernails and skin can shed light on circulation to the extremities, possible vitamin deficiencies, and general health. Skin sensitivity and texture, such as itching or numbness, dryness, wrinkles, or loss of skin tone, may speak to possible fluid and dietary needs. Pay attention to your body's signals! The strength and appearance of your fingernails and the condition and recuperative powers of your skin can be external signs of internal health and nutritional needs.

IS EATING RIGHT ENOUGH?

You want to maintain a healthy diet as a first measure of natural care not just for your hands but also for your entire body. You say you are eating a relatively healthy diet, including a variety of fresh fruits and vegetables that contain natural antioxidants. But do you need vitamin and mineral supplements as well? The answer's not simple and will differ from individual to individual. For example, vitamin D needs go up with age, and calcium requirements dip in the late teens and rise again after age fifty. And not every nutrient that goes in your mouth reaches the cells needing their benefit.

Often overlooked, the oldest, best, and most obvious route to good health is fresh, natural, wholesome food. Nourishment that contains vitamins, minerals, fiber, and juice comes with the most exotic packaging — skins, peels, husks, and rinds. Increasing our consumption of fruits and vegetables to five or more servings a day can significantly reduce the risk of many chronic and life-threatening diseases.

WATER AND THE HUMAN BODY

Even with all of the nutrients available in vitamin and mineral supplements, we cannot afford to overlook the importance of water for our bodily needs. Water is essential to life and is the principal ingredient within all living cells. Almost all of our bodily functions, including digestion, metabolism, respiration, waste removal, and temperature balance, are processed in the presence of — you guessed it — water.

Did you know that a newborn baby's body is 77% water, that children are around 59% water, and that adults are between 45 and 65% water? Our blood is 83% water, our brain is 74% water, our muscles are 75% water, and human bones just 22% water.

Only oxygen is more necessary to sustaining the life of all the inhabitants of this planet. Humans can live about five weeks without protein, carbohydrates, and fats, but in a temperate climate, we can survive only five days without water.

Water circulates perpetually between the blood and bodily organs, dissolving and transporting nutrients, plumping our tissues, augmenting the suppleness of our skin, and maintaining the balance of chemical reactions. But some of our storehouse of water evaporates or is excreted each day and must be replaced.

To replace this lost water, we need to supply our bodies with about three quarts (3 liters) of water through fluids and foods every day. Foods can usually only provide us with about 1½ quarts (1½ liters) of water. The rest, about six glasses' worth, must be supplied by drinking water. Do it. You'll reap the benefits.

But there are other factors to be considered. Today, our foods are grown with an emphasis on mass production. Sprayed with chemicals, injected with hormones, and factory-refined and processed — it's no wonder that the micronutrients essential for health are diminished in our foods. Adding basic vitamin supplements to our diet may be the most efficient way to fulfill the suggested daily nutrient values.

Identifying Nutritional Deficiencies

The absence of an essential vitamin can prevent the completion of normal chemical reactions in the body and will eventually lead to tissue damage. For example, an inadequate amount of vitamin D, needed to assimilate calcium, may lead to porous, weak bones. A deficiency in vitamin A may result in dry, scaly skin, while a lack of B-complex vitamins may account for fingernail problems.

Most often a tissue breakdown involves more than one nutrient, as vitamins usually function in conjunction with each other. Even if your diet is balanced and diverse, certain conditions can still place you at risk for missing nutrients:

Stress. Individuals dealing with stress from illness, infections, or surgery have increased requirements for B-complex, C, and E vitamins.

Dieting. Dieters with low calorie intakes may need multivitamin supplements.

Age. Elders, whose digestive systems tend to absorb fewer vitamins from food, may need multivitamin supplements.

Smoking. Cigarette smokers may have low levels of vitamin C.

Alcohol. Heavy drinkers may need thiamine, riboflavin, folic acid, vitamins B_1, B_2, and C, and more.

Pregnancy. Pregnant women and nursing mothers often need larger amounts of vitamins and minerals.

Women. Women of child-bearing age may need extra iron.

Chronic illness. The chronically ill may be taking medications that deplete nutrients or retard absorption. For example:

- Antibiotics destroy "friendly" intestinal bacteria and lower the body's levels of B-complex vitamins.
- Diuretics can reduce calcium and potassium levels.
- Aspirin and nonsteroidal anti-inflammatory drugs affect levels of vitamin C.
- Corticosteroids can modify vitamins B_6 and C and the mineral zinc.

Nutritional Therapy for Your Hands

Here is a "quick-look" chart of some of the important vitamins and minerals especially beneficial for fingernails, skin, and hands. Use this chart to identify possible vitamin needs according to any concerns or symptoms you may be experiencing. Then turn to the more detailed explanations — what they do, what foods you can find them in, signs of deficiency, and suggested dosages — on the following pages for an in-depth understanding.

QUICK-LOOK VITAMINS AND MINERALS
THAT CAN BENEFIT THE HANDS

A–Z for the Hand	Vitamins and Minerals
Allergic Response	B_5, B_6, C
Arthritis	B_3, B_5, B_6, C, E, calcium, folic acid, selenium, zinc
Blood cells (affecting immune response, skin color)	B_{12}, calcium
Bones	D, calcium
Bruising	C
Burns and sunburn	A, B-complex, C, E
Carpal tunnel	B_6
Circulation to the extremities	B_3, C, E
Collagen, connective tissue	B_1, B_5, B_6
Dermatitis	B_3, B_6, B_{12}
Dry skin	A, B-complex, C, EFA (essential fatty acids)
Eczema	B_5, GLA (gamma-linolenic acids)
Edema	B_6
Fingernail texture and strength	A, B-complex, B_2, biotin, iron, zinc
Fungus infections	A, B-complex, C
Immune system (affecting your response to infection)	B_2, C, E, zinc
Insect bites, stings	C, calcium
Itching	iron
Muscles	B_6
Nervous system	B_1, B_6, B_{12}, magnesium, potassium
Pigmentation of the skin	A, B-complex, C, D, E, folacin
Psoriasis	A, B-complex, C, D, E, folacin, EFAs
Raynaud's phenomenon	C, E, GLA
Scars	E, zinc
Skin	A, B_3, C, E, EFAs
Skin ulcers	C, E, EFAs, folacin
Wrinkles	A, B_1, C, E, selenium, zinc

NUTRITIONAL SUPPLEMENTS FOR HEALTHY HANDS

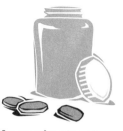

For best absorption and to get those "elephant" pills down, take supplements with food. Capsules are easiest to swallow. If you take vitamins only once a day, take them with or after your largest meal. (Let's hope that's lunch.)

First choice, though, is to replenish these nutrients with real foods in a well-balanced diet. Don't waste precious calories and be vitamin-deficient by stuffing yourself with filling but nutritionally empty junk food. Your body will be a lot happier with carrots, celery, and apples instead of potato chips, candy bars, and diet soda. You are what you eat! (Now, if only I could take my own advice on a regular basis!)

When we do need more nutrients, then it's time to reach for supplements. Vitamin labels list the percentage of the U.S. RDA (Recommended Daily Allowance) or DV (Daily Value) guidelines, but these specifications are for perfectly healthy people. If you have a particular condition or an uneven nutritional lifestyle, you may need higher potencies. Get expert advice before trying to treat specific problems with micronutrients. Look for guidance on the supplements that best meet your needs from a health professional experienced in nutrition and vitamin therapy.

> There is no better seasoning
> for food than laughter.
>
> — Maurice Mességué

Take into account that vitamin therapy does not produce results overnight. Repair or relief can take weeks and sometimes months before the benefits are noticed.

VITAMIN A

Also known as: Retinol

What it is: A fat-soluble vitamin

What it does for the hands: Vitamin A is essential for bone growth and the development of white blood cells. This vitamin speeds healing of wounds and burns and fights infection and skin diseases.

Possible symptoms of deficiency: Fingernails that split, break off, are extremely thin, or fail to grow; decreased ability to see in dim light; or dry, scaly skin.

What foods have it? Vitamin A is found only in foods of animal origin but beta-carotene, its precursor (meaning that it is converted in the body to vitamin A), is found in many fruits and vegetables, including apricots, beet greens, broccoli, cantaloupe, carrots, nectarines, peaches, red peppers, plums, spinach, sweet potatoes, tomatoes, watermelon, and winter squash. Liver and fish-liver oil are also good sources of vitamin A.

Daily supplement dosage: 7,500 to 10,000 IU (international units). Unless you have a specific health condition that demands more, it's best to stay at this level. Consult your healthcare practitioner before increasing the amount of supplement for this vitamin.

Caution: Because vitamin A can accumulate in organ tissues, be cautious of extremely high doses.

THE B-COMPLEX GROUP

The B vitamins maintain nails, skin, hair, eyes, and mucous membranes. There are eleven common B vitamins: thiamine (B_1), riboflavin (B_2), niacin and niacinamide (B_3), pantothenic acid (B_5), pyridoxine (B_6), folic acid (folacin), cyanocobalamin (B_{12}), biotin, para-amino-benzoic acid (PABA), inositol, and choline.

The B vitamins are water-soluble and must be replaced daily. In a supplement, take them together as a B-complex group. A deficiency in one B vitamin may signal a deficiency in another, so a balance needs to be maintained.

VITAMIN B_1

Also known as: Thiamine

What it is: A water-soluble member of the B-complex group

What it does for the hands: Vitamin B_1 helps keep our collagen-rich connective tissues healthy and maintains smooth muscle. B_1 is also necessary for nervous system function and for converting blood sugar into energy. Natural practitioners frequently recommend thiamine for alleviating shingles and neuralgia.

Possible symptoms of deficiency: Memory loss and mental deterioration, numbness, muscle weakness, and tingling in the extremities.

Possible causes of deficiency: Coffee, tea, raw fish, alcohol, and excess sugar can destroy thiamine; a folic acid deficiency can decrease the absorption of thiamine.

What foods have it? Whole grains, brewer's yeast, brown rice, kidney beans, peas, nuts, potatoes, seafood, liver, milk, and lean meats.

Daily supplement dosage: 1 to 1.5 mg

VITAMIN B$_2$

Also known as: Riboflavin

What it is: A water-soluble, B-complex vitamin that sometimes causes bright yellow urine (it's harmless)

What it does for the hands: This vitamin enhances immune function and is necessary for healthy nails and hair.

Possible symptoms of deficiency: Discolored, slightly purplish tongue

Possible causes of deficiency: Oral contraceptives, alcohol, and tobacco diminish the actions of this vitamin.

What foods have it? Brewer's yeast, liver, wheat germ, green vegetables, and legumes.

Daily supplement dosage: 1.2 to 1.7 mg

VITAMIN B$_3$

Also known as: Niacin

What it is: A water-soluble member of the B-complex group

What it does for the hands: Vitamin B$_3$ is effective in improving circulation by dilating blood vessels. It may be helpful for those with Raynaud's phenomenon. It is vital to the proper activity of the nervous system and for the formation and maintenance of healthy skin. Niacinamide, another form of B$_3$, may be helpful for those with osteoarthritis.

Possible symptoms of deficiency: Bad breath, canker sores, insomnia, irritability, depression, recurring headaches, general fatigue, and/or loss of appetite. Severe niacin deficiency results in pellagra, a disease characterized in part by dermatitis, rough inflamed skin, tremors, and nervous disorders.

Possible causes of deficiency: Antibiotics and excessive consumption of sugar and starches will deplete the body's supply of niacin.

What foods have it? Brewer's yeast, whole grains, liver, poultry, fish, milk, wheat bran, green vegetables, and legumes.

Daily supplement dosage: Women should take 13 mg daily; men should take 16 mg. Various illnesses can increase the need for niacin. Larger doses (100 mg or more) of niacin may cause passing side effects such as intense flushing of the skin, tingling, and itching; these symptoms are not usually seen with niacinamide.

Caution: Do not take supplements of niacin if you suffer from peptic ulcers or gout.

VITAMIN B₅

Also known as: Pantothenic acid

What it is: A water-soluble member of the B-complex group

What it does for the hands: Vitamin B₅ helps to prevent premature aging and wrinkles. This may also be a useful vitamin in the treatment of arthritis, allergies, and eczema.

Possible symptoms of deficiency: Deficiencies are rare and difficult to determine because this vitamin is readily available in many foods. Because pantothenic acid helps build antibodies for fighting infection, someone with low levels of B₅ might be susceptible to recurring infections.

Possible causes of deficiency: Methyl bromide, a fumigant in foods, immobilizes this vitamin.

What foods have it? Brewer's yeast, egg yolks, and whole-grain cereals are the richest sources of vitamin B₅.

Daily supplement dosage: 5 to 15 mg; therapeutic doses may be larger.

VITAMIN B₆

Also known as: Pyridoxine

What it is: A water-soluble member of the B-complex group

What it does for the hands: Vitamin B₆ must be present for the production of antibodies and red blood cells. It helps maintain the body's balance of sodium and potassium for normal function of the nervous and musculoskeletal systems. This vitamin has been shown to be of some benefit in treating carpal tunnel syndrome and as an antiallergy supplement.

In one research study, daily B₆ capsules were given to men and women at midlife who had developed painful knots on the sides of their finger joints as a result of osteoarthritis. Joints ceased to be painful, knots reduced in size, and hand flexion improved within six weeks. B_6 injections have also been shown to be of some value to those with Parkinson's disease.

Possible symptoms of deficiency: Low blood sugar and sensitivity to insulin; loss of hair; puffy fingers because of water retention; arthritis; dermatitis; and hand numbness, including such as tingling hands and tingling wrist-to-hand or shoulder-to-hand syndromes.

What foods have it? Meats, whole grains, brewer's yeast, legumes, potatoes, carrots, eggs, and bananas; desiccated liver and brewer's yeast are recommended supplements.

Daily supplement dosage: 10 mg; a therapeutic dosage is 50 to 200 mg. Take B_6 as a supplement with breakfast, as it may cause intense dreams and restlessness if taken at night. The need for B_6 increases during pregnancy and with age. However, check with your healthcare provider before increasing any dosages.

VITAMIN B_{12}

Also known as: Cyanocobalamin

What it is: A water-soluble vitamin of the B-complex group. It is the only vitamin that contains cobalt, an essential mineral element. Like penicillin, B_{12} grows in bacteria or molds.

What it does for the hands: Vitamin B_{12} is required for the formation of red blood cells and the function of a normal nervous system. Reports suggest that vitamin B_{12} may be of value in treating excessive scaling and itching of the skin caused by a disturbance of the sebaceous glands.

Possible symptoms of deficiency: Hand pigmentation in individuals with black skin; major deficiencies of this vitamin could cause changes in the nervous system and difficulty in walking.

Possible causes of deficiency: Those with poor digestive systems may have difficulty absorbing this vitamin. People on vegetarian diets may be low in B_{12} and high in folic acid, which would mask a B_{12} deficiency. The use of laxatives depletes the storage of B_{12}.

What foods have it? Eggs, fish, liver, and kidneys.

Daily supplement dosage: 2 to 3 micrograms for adults. B_6, magnesium, and calcium enable absorption of B_{12} by the body. Absorption of B_{12} is improved when it is taken spaced over several meals.

BIOTIN

What it is: A water-soluble member of the B-complex group. This essential nutrient appears in trace amounts in all animal and plant tissue.

What it does for the hands: Biotin is a sulfur-containing organic compound involved in the metabolism of fatty acids. In recent clinical studies, biotin was shown to thicken and hydrate nails and make them less brittle or susceptible to splitting and cracking.

Possible symptoms of deficiency: Dermatitis, grayish skin color, dry skin, and sleeplessness.

Possible causes of deficiency: Deficiency states seem to occur when the diet consists of too many egg whites. Oral antibiotics may also cause a biotin deficiency by destroying the intestinal bacteria necessary for synthesis of this vitamin. If you must be on antibiotics, protect your tummy by eating nonfat or low-fat yogurt with active cultures. Buy an organic brand that specifies the live active yogurt cultures, that is, *Lactobacillus acidophilus*, *L. bulgaricus*, *Streptococcus thermophilus*, or *S. bifidus.*

What foods have it? Bananas, cauliflower, mushrooms, unpolished rice, brewer's yeast, fish, legumes (such as peanuts and lentils), and dairy products.

Daily supplement dosage: 150 to 300 micrograms

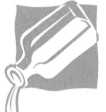

VITAMIN C

Also known as: Ascorbic acid or ascorbate

What it is: A water-soluble nutrient with a wide range of benefits

What it does for the hands: This vitamin is an essential building block in the manufacture and repair of collagen, a protein necessary for the formation of connective tissue in skin and bones. Vitamin C also helps to stimulate skin cells to produce new tissue in the scars of wounds and burns. It also aids in reducing the wrinkling and sagging skin that occurs with aging.

Arthritis sufferers should note that studies show the lubricating fluid of joints (synovial fluid) becomes thinner (for ease of movement) when blood levels of ascorbic acid are high.

Powdered vitamin C mixed with water to form a paste and applied to the skin is a treatment for spider bites, insect stings, and poison ivy, along with simultaneous oral doses.

In various research studies dealing with the body's ability to adjust to heat and cold, vitamin C supplements (500 to 2000 mg per day) have been shown to help our internal body thermostats adjust to changes in temperature at both ends of the scale. This may become an important vitamin for those with Raynaud's phenomenon or those venturing into very cold climates and worried about frostbite.

Possible symptoms of deficiency: Bleeding gums, tendency to bruising, swollen or painful joints, and slow healing of wounds and fractures. Severe lack of vitamin C results in scurvy.

Possible causes of deficiency: The body's ability to absorb this vitamin is reduced by smoking, stress, high fever, antibiotics, cortisone, and aspirin. Cooking foods in copper pots destroys their vitamin C content.

What foods have it? Asparagus, bananas, cantaloupe, citrus fruits, broccoli, brussels sprouts, cabbage, cauliflower, green and red peppers, potatoes, squash, and tomatoes.

Daily supplement dosage: The US RDA for vitamin C is 200 mg, although most supplements contain considerably more than that. Since most vitamin C is out of the body in three or four hours, in order to maintain an adequate level you should take small doses throughout the day. For therapeutic doses, take 250 to 500 mg three times a day. The need for vitamin C increases with age.

Cautions: Vitamin C supplements may affect sugar-level tests in diabetics and tests for blood in stools. Very high doses may also cause abdominal cramps and a loose stool.

CALCIUM

What it is: The most abundant mineral in the body, found primarily in our bones and teeth

What it does for the hands: Calcium is essential for healthy blood and bones. It acts with phosphorus to build and maintain bony tissue.

Possible causes of deficiency: These foods, along with a sedentary lifestyle, leech calcium from our bones: sugar, caffeine, excessive protein, excessive alcohol, and the phosphates found in soda.

What foods have it? Leafy green vegetables, such as kale and collard greens; fortified orange juice; tofu made with calcium sulfate, low-fat yogurt or skim milk; sardines with soft bones; and salmon.

Daily supplement dosage: Supplement with calcium ascorbate or calcium citrate to equal 1000 mg daily from ages nineteen to fifty. If you are over fifty, increase the amount to at least 1200 mg. Check the label for the amount of pure or "elemental" calcium in each tablet — this tells you the usable amount. Stay away from bonemeal, oyster shell, and dolomite. Calcium is most beneficial when taken with milk or yogurt, between meals and before bed.

Those taking 1500 mg of calcium daily should add 10 mg of supplemental zinc. Studies show that this much calcium a day interferes with zinc absorption and balance. It's not simple — one thing affects another.

Hint: Take time out from your calcium supplements one week every three months to give your body time to signal the need for natural bone remodeling. Increase your amount of weight-bearing exercise during this time.

VITAMIN D

What it is: A fat-soluble vitamin normally obtained from sunshine. When you understand how vitamin D works, you can appreciate the interrelationship of our health to the environment. The sun's rays on the skin trigger a biochemical reaction for vitamin D production. With just 10 minutes a day in the sun, your body will be able to manufacture its own vitamin D supply.

What it does for the hands: This vitamin helps the body maintain its balance of calcium, which is essential for healthy bones and blood. We can't produce our own calcium but must get it from the food we eat. Vitamin D, formed in the skin, is converted by the body to a hormone called calciferol. This hormone moves calcium to the skeleton through the bloodstream. When the body doesn't get enough vitamin D, the bones don't get calcium, nor do other parts of the body.

Vitamin D, as calciferol, tells our intestines when to absorb more calcium from the food we eat. If we are not getting enough calcium in our food, vitamin D orders the body to remove calcium from our bones!

Possible symptoms of deficiency: Soft or brittle bones. A vitamin D deficiency causes a calcium deficiency (even with calcium supplements), and thus bone loss.

Since sunscreens with an SPF of 8 prevent 95 percent of our skin's production of vitamin D, spend 10 to 15 minutes walking outside in the sunlight, *without sunscreen,* two to three times a week. (If you are very sun sensitive, high noon may not be the best time for your little bit of sunlight. However, the best hours are between 8 A.M. and 4 P.M.) During this outside time, expose your hands, face, and arms to the sun.

To test for a vitamin D deficiency, ask your doctor for a 25-hydroxyvitamin D test.

What foods have it? Cod-liver oil and some fatty fish such as kippers are natural sources of vitamin D. The only food that is fortified with vitamin D, at present, is milk — other dairy products do not contain this vitamin.

Daily supplement dosage: After the age of fifty, take a 400 to 600 IU vitamin D supplement every day. After age seventy, the D supplement should be raised to 800 IU a day. (Do not take more than 1000 IU of vitamin D a day from all sources.)

Cautions: Not all cases of osteoporosis respond well to increased vitamin D. Postmenopausal women, with a reduced production of body estrogen, may find that their bodies have some interference with the conversion of vitamin D to its hormonal form, so their bones are deprived of calcium. Also, some drugs and vitamin D interfere with each other. Check with your healthcare provider if you are bothered by symptoms of bone tenderness, pain, or weakness.

VITAMIN E

What it is: A fat-soluble vitamin. Vitamin E is an antioxidant, which means it opposes oxidation of substances in the body and helps eliminate free radicals that damage cells.

What it does for the hands: This vitamin helps maintain healthy circulation and improves the efficiency of the body's oxygen use. Because vitamin E somewhat delays the formation of collagen, applying it to a wound, skin ulcers, or abrasions keeps the skin from overcontracting as it heals and helps to produce thinner, more flexible scars. Vitamin E can also relieve the itching of dry skin.

Possible symptoms of deficiency: Loss of reflex response; another clinical sign is the breakdown of red blood cells.

Possible causes of deficiency: Female estrogen is a vitamin E antagonist.

What foods have it? Cold-pressed vegetable oils, wheat germ oil, raw seeds and nuts, and soybeans.

Daily supplement dosage: 400 IU; the best time to take vitamin E is after a meal or at bedtime. Chlorine destroys vitamin E in the body, so if you have chlorinated drinking water, filter it if you can. Initial intake should be low and gradually increased; vitamin E has a tendency to raise blood pressure.

Caution: Those with chronic rheumatic heart disease should check with their physician before starting vitamin E therapy.

FOLIC ACID

What it is: A water-soluble member of the B-complex group

What it does for the hands: Folic acid functions as a coenzyme with vitamins B_{12} and C in the breakdown and use of proteins in the body. It is essential for the production of red blood cells. There is some evidence that daily supplements of folate will benefit those with osteoarthritis of the hands and those with psoriasis.

Possible symptoms of deficiency: Sometimes what looks like an iron deficiency is actually a lack of folate. (Folate is one form of folic acid.) Anemia can occur when there is not enough folate in the body to produce red blood cells.

What foods have it? Dark green, leafy vegetables; liver; and brewer's yeast.

Daily supplement dosage: Around 400 micrograms per day. Pregnant or nursing women should increase their folate intake to 600 to 800 micrograms (check first with your healthcare provider). High doses (5 mg) are presently available only by prescription.

Caution: An excessive intake of folic acid can mask a vitamin B_{12} deficiency.

GAMMA-LINOLENIC ACID (GLA)

What it is: A polyunsaturated fatty acid that promotes the healthy growth of skin and nails. It also is an effective anti-inflammatory agent.

What it does for the hands: Gamma-linolenic acid maintains healthy tissues by regulating the moisture balance of the skin, nails, and hair. GLA capsules are sometimes recommended for the treatment of arthritis; soft or brittle fingernails; acne; dry, wrinkled skin; and eczema. It may take six to eight weeks to notice benefits from this supplement.

What foods have it? GLA is naturally present in mother's milk and is formed in the body from linoleic acid. Sources of GLA are found in the seed oils of evening primrose, borage, black currant, as well as sunflower and gooseberry seeds.

Daily supplement dosage: Depending on the source of GLA, the dosage will differ:

Evening primrose oil: A fatty oil obtained from the small seeds of evening primrose. Take 500 mg with 40 mg of GLA; two to six capsules/day. (*Caution:* Not recommended for those with epilepsy.)

Borage oil: An oil obtained from the seeds of the borage plant. Take 1000 mg with 240 mg of GLA; 1 capsule per day. (*Caution:* If you are planning to take borage oil over an extended period of time, look for products that are free of UPAs [unsaturated pyrrolizidine alkaloids]. Borage contains low levels of UPAs, which have been found responsible for a disease of the veins of the liver known as veno-occlusive disease.)

Black currant oil: An oil obtained from the seeds of black currant. Take 500 mg with 80 mg GLA per capsule; three per day.

In making the choice, Dr. Andrew Weil, a well-known proponent of natural medicine, suggests that the seeds of black currants are twice as rich in gamma-linolenic acid as is evening primrose oil. But it is easier to take only one capsule a day with borage oil. To boost results, add leafy green vegetables, raisins, and whole grains to your diet.

Caution: Some of the commercially available GLA products may be adulterated with cheaper oils such as soy or safflower. Always buy from a reputable source.

IRON

What it is: An essential part of our blood that is present in every living cell. All iron exists in the body in combination with protein.

What it does for the hands: Iron combines with protein and copper in making hemoglobin, the coloring matter of red blood cells. Hemoglobin transports oxygen and carbon dioxide throughout the body.

Possible symptoms of deficiency: Pale dry skin; spoon-shaped, brittle nails; and, if severe, bleeding into the skin.

Possible causes of deficiency: The most common deficiency of iron is iron deficiency anemia, in which the amount of hemoglobin in the red blood cells is reduced.

What foods have it? Dried apricots, dates, prunes, and raisins; beet greens and spinach; lentils and nuts; peas, lima beans, and chickpeas; eggs; and organ meats such as liver and tongue.

Daily supplement dosage: If a clinical test shows low levels of iron, supplements of ferrous fumarate in a timed-release 50-mg tablet may be a good choice. Ask your doctor. Absorption of iron is improved when taken with vitamin C supplements or with foods rich in vitamin C, such as oranges.

Caution: Excessive deposits of iron can occur from a diseased state of the liver and from diabetes.

SILICON

What it is: An essential trace mineral. The most abundant elements in the earth's crust are a network of oxygen and silicon atoms — oxygen makes up 46 percent of the crust and silicon about 28 percent. Silicon does not occur naturally in a free state but is found in compounds such as silica or silicon dioxide.

What it does for the hands: Silicon is a component of connective tissue and a factor in the strength and elasticity of bone cartilage. Silica in the diet or as a supplement helps to prevent osteoporosis as well as strengthens our fingernails and toenails.

Possible causes of deficiency: Aging and low estrogen levels impair the body's ability to absorb silica.

What foods have it? The best sources of silicon are vegetables, especially the skins of organically grown radishes; whole grains, like oats and alfalfa; and seafood. Horsetail tea, made from one of the richest plant sources of this mineral, is another way to obtain silica (for the tea recipe, see page 69). You can also purchase silica gel from natural food and health stores.

Daily supplement dosage: Take 1 tablespoon of silica gel daily in tea or water to help prevent fingernail breakage.

ZINC

What it is: An essential trace mineral occurring in the body.

What it does for the hands: Supplements of zinc encourage the healing of burns and wounds, enhance immune function, and help treat acne and other skin disorders.

Possible symptoms of deficiency: A zinc deficiency is a factor in stress, fatigue, susceptibility to infection, injury, decreased alertness, and prolonged healing of wounds. Stretch marks in the skin, brittle nails, and white spots in the fingernails could also be due to a lack of zinc.

Possible causes of deficiency: The most common cause of zinc deficiency is an unbalanced diet.

What foods have it? Whole-grain products, brewer's yeast, wheat bran, wheat germ, and pumpkin seeds.

Daily supplement dosage: The usual dose is in the form of zinc gluconate, which is well absorbed when taken as 30 mg of zinc along with 3 mg of copper for balance. (Remember to take 10 mg of zinc daily if you are taking 1500 mg of calcium a day.)

Caution: Nausea and vomiting may be symptoms of zinc overdose.

HEALTHY STRUMMIN' NAILS

Toronto's George Jamieson, a well-known guitarist, in an article in *Guitar Player* magazine, recommends sunscreen to harden nails. Jamieson applies liquid silica to his nails in the form of any "sweatproof" sunscreen with silica. When the sunscreen dries, he "slathers" hair conditioner (a rich one for damaged hair) on top. He claims the silica helps absorb the conditioner and keeps his nails strong and supple. Jamieson uses the sunscreen remedy twice a week and the conditioner daily. If you have weak or soft nails, you might want to give this remedy a try.

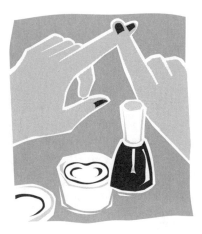

Starting at the Tips: Caring for Your Fingernails

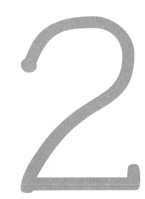

PART 2

CHAPTER 4
Fingernail Diagnostics:
A Window to Healthy Nails

Were it not for the fingers, the hand would be a spoon.

— African proverb

How many times during a day are your fingernails in use? Tell me about the itchy spot on your arm. Did you scratch it? And the dirty spot on the counter? Was it scraped away with the edge of a fingernail? Did you separate a sticky label from its backing or remove a staple with your nails? Our fingernails are truly our first tools. They help us manipulate fine objects and care for ourselves, and are a unique site for personal adornment.

In everyday life, our extremely "handy" fingernails are most conspicuous for how they decorate us. But whether fingernails receive credit for augmenting our appearance or for their convenience and service, it's worthwhile to know how to take care of them. Once you understand the basics, it will be easy to have and maintain healthy nails for the rest of your life.

WHAT MAKES A FINGERNAIL?

Probably the only time we focus on our fingernails is when we break or chip one and have to repair it. But nails offer us more than a fashion statement. Why do we have fingernails? A major responsibility of nails is shielding the delicate nerve endings at the tips of our fingers. Fingernails also contribute to the precision and sensation of touch, enhancing our dexterity and aiding the fingers in grasping objects. Our nails harbor the sensations of touch, temperature, and pain.

Nail Matrix

Nail growth begins in the nail matrix. Like human hair, the hard plate of fingernails is composed of a tough protein called keratin. Matrix cells make the keratin that becomes the visible, strong fingernail. The nail matrix, where the matrix cells collect, contains the nerves, lymph vessels, and blood vessels vital for nourishing the fingernails.

Nail Bed and Nail Plate

The nail bed is, appropriately enough, the bed of skin on which the nail plate and nail matrix rest. As keratin forms in the nail matrix, it pushes further forward onto the nail bed to harden and become the exposed nail plate (the clear shield commonly thought of as the fingernail). The tough nail plate contains none of the nerves or blood vessels found in the nail bed. It's no longer living tissue. Although the nail plate appears to be one solid piece, it is actually constructed in layers. You may notice these layers when a fingernail splits.

The record for having the world's longest nails is currently held by a woman in India. Picture fingernails that range in length from 40 to 52 inches (100 to 130 cm). That's 3 to 5 feet (90 to 150 cm) long! Imagine trying to take care of an itch!

For all they are able to do, it is surprising that normal nails are only $1/50$ of an inch thick. When the nails are healthy, the nail plate remains firmly attached to the nail bed and continues to grow. Nail growth is dependent on good nutrition and general wellness.

Nail Fold

This layer of skin covers the edges of the nail plate on all sides except the tip, and holds the nail in place. It is often the primary site of nail fungus infections.

Cuticles

The cuticle, a small piece of skin that sometimes overhangs the nail plate, is one of the most important parts of the nail. The cuticle protects the nail matrix, the delicate tissues and cells below the nail plate that are actively forming the hard nail.

Any vigorous pushing back of the cuticles, trimming, or chemical solvents will cause ridges in the nail. And worse than ridges, once the cuticle is damaged, the watertight space under

LOVE YOUR CUTICLES!

Don't be swayed by fashion trends. Cuticles on the nails are necessary, normal, and okay. Don't cut your cuticles; they are there for the protection of your growing nail. If you feel that your cuticles are rough or unsightly, treat them with a demulcent nail soak and moisturizing cuticle oils. (For more information on caring for your cuticles, see chapter 6, beginning on page 78.)

the nail fold is open to moisture and becomes a potential breeding ground for bacteria, yeast infections, and deformed nails. (One such condition is called boggy finger; see pages 188–190 for a description and suitable remedies.)

Moons

We know that the birth of the fingernail takes place under the all-important cuticle. The milky white crescent formed at the base of the nail, crossed by the cuticle, is the half-moon, or lunula. This is a semi-transparent window to the nail matrix and nail bed underneath. The lunula is easiest to see on the thumb and hardest to see on the little finger. It may sometimes be obscured by the cuticle.

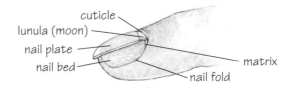

cuticle
lunula (moon)
nail plate
nail bed
matrix
nail fold

NAIL GROWTH

Fingernails wear down with use. Good biological planning arranged for nails to grow constantly during life. But there are variables that can affect how nails grow and nail growth, in turn, can offer information about your health and diet.

Following are some fingernail facts that you can use to impress your friends:

◆ Nail growth is different from person to person and from finger to finger. If your nails grow quickly, this is one measure that you are well nourished. Conversely, nails grow more slowly if you are ill or have a poor diet. In most cases, the nail on the middle finger grows the fastest and the nail on the little finger grows the slowest.

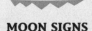

MOON SIGNS

It's been theorized that the size, shape, and color of finger-nail "moons" are inherited. Compare the moons on your fingers to those of your family. Are they similar or different? Lunulas that seem large for the nail may be an indication of an overactive thyroid gland. Not having moons on any of the nails may indicate an underactive thyroid gland or could be normal. Both of these "moon" conditions can be genetic and offer clues to a familial predisposition to certain health problems. Thyroid hormones stimulate the body's protein synthesis, oxygen consumption, and cell division and thereby affect the epidermis (the outer layer of skin). The effects of thyroid disease on the nails is still poorly understood, but the thyroid gland has a definite role in keratin production cycles of the hair and skin.

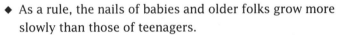

- ◆ As a rule, the nails of babies and older folks grow more slowly than those of teenagers.
- ◆ The length of the finger and the size of its moon suggest the speed of growth of the nail. The shorter the finger and the less of its visible moon, the more slowly the nail will grow. (The thumb is the exception.)
- ◆ Biting fingernails, while detrimental to their health in other ways, is thought to make them grow faster.
- ◆ Fingernails grow faster than toenails, and all nails grow more quickly in summer than in winter or cold weather. Heat increases the rate of all metabolic processes.
- ◆ Nails grow faster during the day than at night due to the natural pulse of body rhythms.
- ◆ Men's nails grow faster than women's. However, women will experience a spurt in nail growth just before menstruation and during pregnancy. These growth spurts are thought to be in response to hormonal activity.

NAIL NUTRITION

To keep fingernails healthy and strong, eat a healthy diet, including vitamin- and mineral-rich foods. Key vitamins and minerals for the nails are vitamins A, B-complex, C, D, E, iron, calcium, magnesium, zinc, sulfur, and essential fatty acids (EFA).

Remember, these elements, taken only as supplements, will be ineffective unless they are part of a varied, healthy diet. Nails grow slowly, so it will be at least three to four months into a fortified diet before you begin to see improvement in the quality of your nails.

FINGERNAIL DIAGNOSTICS

As early as 400 B.C.E., Hippocrates taught that the nails reflect the condition of the inner body. It is true that abnormalities of the nails can often provide early clues to common medical problems or severe systemic diseases.

We see color in the natural nail, but the fingernail itself is colorless and translucent. The central portion of the normal nail appears pink because the nail bed below the nail plate is rich in capillaries, and the nail plate is close-fitting. The free edge of the nail is white because of air beneath it. The lunula, or moon, appears white because it is not firmly attached to the nail plate.

But life can have an impact on our fingernails, changing their texture, hardness, color, thickness, and shape. These changes are worth noting because they speak to us of our inner health.

Lines and Ridges on the Fingernails

Take a few moments and examine your unpolished fingernails under a good light. You will gather a new appreciation for how your lifestyle affects your nails and overall health.

Long lines. As people age, longitudinal lines appear in the nails. These long lines are not considered important, and we know of no way to prevent them. Think of these lines as age wrinkles on the nails. (You'd have thought we would be safe from wrinkles somewhere on our bodies!)

There is some new thinking that long, corrugated lines on the nails may be due to the body's poor absorption of vitamins and minerals, or that these nail lines may signal anemia. More research is needed in this area. Some nutrients, in food and supplements, seem to be especially important in general nail health, including vitamins A, B-complex, and C, as well as calcium, magnesium, zinc, and essential fatty acids.

White lines. White lines across the nail bed are common, but sometimes are indications of liver or kidney disease.

Ridges. Any inflammation or irritation around the area of the nail matrix disturbs the growth pattern of the nail plate, and a lengthwise furrow is produced. Cuticle manipulation, such as cutting too much of the cuticle or pushing it back too vigorously, can cause fingernail ridging.

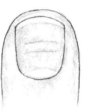

Beau's lines — horizontal ridges that cross the nail like wavy furrows — indicate that something has interrupted nail growth, such as high fever, nutritional deficiencies, drug reactions, painful menstruation, childbirth, or trauma from surgery. The nail matrix stops producing keratin. When the nail begins to grow again, a groove marks the spot where the nail-forming cells rested.

CLOCKING NAIL INJURIES

Nails grow at different rates due to age, nutrition, and health factors. Under the best of conditions, a nail grows about 0.004 inches (0.1 mm) a day or 1/8 of an inch (3 mm) each month. It takes about six months for a new nail to grow from cuticle to tip. If you're the scientific type, you can estimate the number of days since an illness or a trauma to the nail by measuring the distance from the horizontal ridge to the cuticle, or proximal nail fold. If the boo-boo occurred near the cuticle in January, it should be growing out by June.

Normal, healthy nails can grow in a variety of shapes, determined by a person's genetics. When we think about everyday fingernail problems, we most often focus on soft or brittle nails and split or pitted nails. These conditions are generally related to the effects of the environment, nail-biting, age, or heredity. However, changes in our nails can also be a signal of other internal health problems, and nail disorders can result from a variety of causes. The following chart outlines some common conditions to watch for.

NAIL DIAGNOSTICS

Nail Condition	Potential Cause
Complete loss of nail	Trauma to the nail; a form of dermatitis; syphilis
Nail plate loose	Injury; nail psoriasis; fungal or bacterial infections; medicines; chemotherapy; thyroid disease; Raynaud's phenomenon; lupus
Wasting away of nails; nail loses luster and becomes smaller	Injury or disease
Thickened nail plate	Poor circulation; fungal infection; heredity; mild, persistent trauma to the nail
Pitted nails sometimes with yellow-to-brown "oil" spots	Eczema or psoriasis; hair loss condition
Very soft nails	Contact with strong alkali; malnutrition; endocrine problems; chronic arthritis

Nail Condition	Potential Cause
Spoon-shaped nails	Iron deficiency; thyroid disease
Clublike nails growing around swollen finger ends	Chronic respiratory or heart problems; cirrhosis of the liver
Horizontal ridges	Injury; infection; nutrition
Longitudinal ridges	Aging; poor absorption of vitamins and minerals; thyroid disease; kidney failure
Brittle, split nails	Nail dryness; nails in contact with irritating substances (detergents, chemicals, polish remover); silica deficiency
Infected nails: red tender, swollen, pus	Bacterial or yeast infection
Overlarge moons	Overactive thyroid; genetics; self-induced trauma (habit tick)
No moons	Underactive thyroid; genetics

Discolored Fingernails

Normally, the color of fingernails is uniform and of a lighter tone than the skin on the back of the hand. The nail bed will show a pinkish color through the nail plate for the fair-skinned and a creamy beige for darker skin tones.

Discolored nails can give clues to internal body imbalances. If you notice an unexplained change in the color of your nails, it could be a sign of a health problem warranting a visit to your doctor. Toxicity to certain medications can also discolor nails.

- **Colorless** fingernails that appear much paler than the surrounding skin may indicate anemia.
- **Red or deep pink** fingernails can indicate a tendency to poor peripheral circulation.
- **Blue** nails may be a sign that the blood is not receiving adequate oxygen due to respiratory disorders, cardio-vascular problems, or lupus erythematosus. Blue nails may also be a reaction to dyes or chemicals.
- **Yellow** nails may be the consequence of colored nail enamels, nail hardeners, tetracycline, fungus, diabetes, psoriasis, or heredity.
- **White, crumbly, soft** nails can result from a fungal infection leading to thickening and ridging of the finger-nails. The fungus usually begins at the free edge of the nail and works its way down to the root.
- **Half white/half pink** nails may indicate a fungal infection or, more seriously, kidney disease.
- **Small white patches** that gradually move down the nail are usually a sign of injury to the nail matrix (such as bending the nail tip too far back) or of contact exposure to harsh soaps or cleaning products.
- **Purple or black** nails are usually due to trauma to the nail (hit the iron nail next time, not your keratin one!) or may also be a sign of vitamin B_{12} deficiency. However, a brown or black streak that begins at the base of the nail and extends to its tip could be a diagnostic clue to a potentially dangerous melanoma. See your healthcare provider to distinguish these streaks from a more serious medical problem.

CHAPTER 5
Common Nail Problems
and Everyday Remedies

Only one thing can bring about
fresh change — new information!

— Anonymous

We rely on our fingernails for so many tasks that periodic maintenance is a must. This care can work to both prevent and relieve many common fingernail problems, such as nail- and cuticle-biting; bacterial, yeast, and fungal infections; and brittle or split nails. If done with care, this time spent may actually be enjoyable.

You can relieve or cure many fingernail problems with simple homemade natural remedies. However, for serious nail infections or lingering ailments, consult with a specialist first — it's a visit of value to prevent chronic, long-term fingernail problems.

NAIL- AND CUTICLE-BITING

"Don't bite the hand that feeds you." Nail-biters' nails are usually short and frayed, but the truth is that biting fingernails is thought to make them grow faster. This may often go unnoticed because nail-biters spend a great deal of time gnawing off fragments of past biting efforts.

Nail-biting and cuticle-biting sometimes go hand-in-hand. It's a difficult behavior to control but one worth changing, as it commonly causes deformed nails, raggedness, infection, hangnails, and warts. Stress — and how we deal with it — is often a factor in this habit. Sigmund Freud theorized that nail-biters are seeking satisfaction of some unfulfilled desire (probably the desire to have healthy, attractive nails and cuticles!). Whatever the reason, following are some tips on how to change this behavior and care for its destructive effects on fingernails.

NAIL-BITERS'
ALOE VERA OINTMENT

For as long as I can remember, I've heard tales of the old-fashioned remedy of coating the nails with a bad-tasting liquid polish. However, I have talked to numerous habitual nail-biters who have grown to love this bitter polish concoction.

A worthy alternative to the chemical polish product is a natural ointment made from the gel of fresh aloe vera leaves.

Several fresh leaves of the aloe vera plant

AMAZING ALOE

According to legend, aloe was one of the plants that grew in the Garden of Eden. This succulent, native to Africa, has a traditional use for healing wounds and as an antifungal agent. A multifunctional plant used for a wide range of basic first-aid purposes, its leaf produces a gel that is helpful for treating sunburn, wrinkles, insect bites, skin irritations, scarring, and minor cuts and scratches.

To cultivate aloe, plant in full sun. Water regularly, but allow the soil to dry out between waterings. In temperate climates, you can grow aloe in a sunny window.

To make:
1. Cut a fresh aloe leaf down the center. With a spoon, scoop out the gel.
2. When you have collected a quantity of gel, place it in a double boiler. Boil the "sticky stuff" down to a thicker, pastelike consistency.
3. Spoon into a small clean jar with lid. Label, date, and store in a cool place.

To use:
When the urge arises to nibble on your fingernails, rub the aloe paste on the edges of the nails. The taste should discourage you.

Caution: A little bit of this gel goes a long way. Large internal doses of concentrated aloe can cause vomiting. If you are pregnant and think you might be tempted to nibble despite the application of ointment, avoid this remedy, as the plant's anthraquinone glycosides are purgative.

For infected nails: Try a warm compress of fresh aloe vera gel. Squeeze the gel directly on the infected finger and cover with a warm, slightly damp cotton cloth.

Caring for Your Hangnails

Hangnails, fleshy bits of dry skin that have split away from the edges of the fingernail, are very common in nail-biters. They can be painful and become a site for secondary infections. Children often have hangnails. This is a good time to give them some direction on how to keep their skin and nails fit. Suggest that they resist the temptation to tear off a hangnail. If it's in the way, cut the flap of skin at its base with clippers or small scissors. Store a bottle or tube of hand cream at every sink and try to get the family in the habit of using it after hand washing. Hangnails can also signal dry cuticles caused by frequent hand washing, cold weather, or rough working conditions. Moisturize the nails and skin around them often. Regularly moisturizing the cuticle area will help cut down on the urge to bite.

Nail Tips, or Caps, for Nail-Biters

In the old days, the remedy for biting nails was a piece of red flannel tied around the most bitten fingers. Today, a more cosmetically appealing alternative is nail tips, or caps, applied to thicken the nail edges. Nail tips are synthetic white nail edges that are tailored to have a natural nail width and arch. They are applied with a coat of adhesive to the free edge of the fingernail. This change in density at the nail point seems to alert nail-biters to reconsider their actions.

If the aloe ointment isn't working, you might want to try a nail-tips remedy for three months. It may be just enough to change the nail-biting habit and relieve the possibility of continual infections around the nails.

Caution: Never apply an artificial nail if the tissue around the natural nail is infected or irritated. Wait until this area is completely healed. Then permit a month's rest for your nails after each three-month period with synthetic nails.

MORE TIME-TESTED IDEAS TO CURB NAIL-BITING

- Sit on your hands when you have the urge to bite your fingernails.
- Clench your fists for a minute.
- Put moisture back — apply cuticle and nail cream as often as you wash your hands.
- Carry a low-grit nail file to smooth rough edges.
- Wear gloves.
- Try acupuncture, hypnotism, or behavioral therapy.

Regular Manicures

Regular home or salon manicures can also help you to break the nail-biting habit. Having attractive hands may act as an incentive to use those "pearly whites" (teeth, that is) for something other than shaping fingernails. (See chapter 6, "The Best Manicure," beginning on page 78.)

NAIL INFECTIONS

Chronic infection of the skin around a fingernail can be due to many causes and is always an uncomfortable condition. A new medical term you may hear is *paronychia,* but the problem has probably bothered folks since caveperson days. An older name for this condition is *whitlow.* Whatever the name, the definition is the same: a break in the skin resulting in a painful inflammation and infection of a finger or toe, directly behind the cuticle or around the nail fold. The area is usually tender, swollen, red, and infected. Pus may be noticeable.

Paronychia can be caused by a bacterial (*Staphylococcus aureus* or *Streptococcus*) or yeast (*Candida*) infection that attacks growing tissue at the base of the nails. The nail plate may show white, rippled, horizontal lines, called Beau's lines, which mark a temporary disturbance in the nail's growth. Thumb-suckers, nail-biters, and nail- or cuticle-pickers are prone to this condition.

If you have an infected nail, visit a dermatologist to have the type of infection analyzed (yeast vs. bacterial), as this will help you get the appropriate treatment. Depending on the cause, remedies could include antibacterial or antifungal agents.

Vitamin Therapy

At the first sign of a nail or skin infection, reach for some helpful vitamins to take daily with meals until the problem has been resolved. I take B-complex vitamins, essential for natural cortisone production — folic acid, niacin, biotin, and 100 to 300 mg pantothenic acid — one-third dose with each meal, plus vitamin C (up to 1000 mg a day). Vitamin C stimulates the production of antibodies and speeds the healing process.

Herbal Remedies

There are also several soothing herbal preparations you can use to treat fingernail infections. As with all ailments, if the problem seems especially serious or is persistent, check in with a specialist or physician for treatment or advice.

WARM FLOWER SOAK

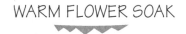

This infusion of lavender or chamomile will help soothe and reduce skin irritations and inflammation. Lavender also helps inhibit bacteria.

1 quart (1 liter) clear soft water or distilled water
2 ounces (60 g) dried German chamomile or lavender flowers
1 teaspoon (5 ml) essential oils of rosemary, lavender, grapefruit, or geranium (optional)

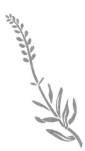

To make:
1. Boil the water and pour, still steaming, over the dried herbs.
2. Steep the flowers in a covered pot (about 20–30 minutes).
3. When the water has cooled to a comfortable temperature, strain the flowers and pour some of the liquid into a small bowl. Or, if you like, save the blossoms and let your fingers play with them while they are immersed in this infusion. If desired, add the essential oils, using any single oil or combination.

To use:
Soak the infected finger for at least 10 minutes, two or three times a day. If you like, re-warm to a comfortable temperature each time you do a soak.
Note: Save the remaining, unused liquid in a closed container in the refrigerator for the next dip; it will keep for about two weeks.
Caution: Those with ragweed allergies may be sensitive to chamomile blossoms.

ANTISEPTIC SOAK

For nail infections that are not healing readily, this regimen may be an alternative approach until you can see your healthcare provider.

1 tablespoon (15 ml) bleach

A few drops mild liquid soap

2 quarts (2 liters) soft water

To make:

1. Boil the water and add the bleach and the liquid soap.

2. Stir with a wooden spoon.

3. Pour 1 cup of this mixture into a small glass bowl and cool to a comfortable temperature.

4. Bottle and label the remaining liquid.

To use:

1. Soak the infected finger three times a day for 10 minutes. You might want to gently warm the bottled liquid in a warm-water bath each time.

2. Repeat this procedure for four days (or longer if the wound has not healed).

PROTECTING NAIL INFECTIONS

When you have an infection around your nails, wear protective gloves to do wet work on such tasks as washing dishes, cars, laundry, and gardening. Turn the gloves inside out and wash them at least once a week. When the infection is gone, toss the gloves. (It's akin to changing your toothbrush after the flu.) For more about gloves, see "If the Glove Fits, Wear It," beginning on page 100.

VERBENA COMPRESS

From the twelfth century, here is Saint Hildegard of Bingen's Verbena Remedy for soothing a whitlow (an infected nail).

Vervain, also known as verbena, has been associated with magic since the time of the Druids. Pliny, A.D. 77, wrote that "people who have been rubbed with it will obtain their wishes, banish fever . . . and cure all disease." With that kind of endorsement, this herb belongs in everyone's garden. Verbena is an astringent and aids in the healing of open wounds.

1 tablespoon (15 ml) verbena leaves and flowers, dried and ground
Spring water to cover

To make:

1. With mortar and pestle, pound the dried verbena to break out its essence.
2. Place the crushed verbena in a small muslin sack with a drawstring. Drop into boiling water and boil for 3 minutes.
3. Press the excess water from the sack and place the muslin with the warm herb on a small, clean, ironed piece of linen large enough to cover the infected finger.

To use:

Wrap the cloth with the herb-filled sack around the finger and leave this compress on until the sack loses its heat. Repeat as needed.

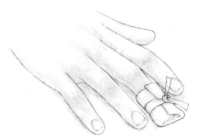

LEMON FOLK REMEDY

In addition to relieving the pain of infection, this treatment will remove stains from your nails. A bonus is that lemon juice restores the natural pH of your skin.

1 or 2 fresh lemons

To use:

1. Cut a small opening at the end of a lemon and push in the affected finger.

2. Keep the infected finger in place until the lemon ceases to draw (stops stinging). If you wish, apply another lemon until the pain is relieved.

Note: If the infection or inflammation continues for a time, the nail will lose luster and have ridges, and the developing nail will be affected. When home remedies don't work, it's time to consult a dermatologist who specializes in nail problems.

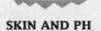

SKIN AND PH

The abbreviation pH stands for "potential hydrogen," but it is commonly used to measure the alkalinity or acidity of a substance. A pH of 7.0 is the neutral point; the neutral range is considered to be 6.5 to 7.5. Water and blood are usually in the neutral range. Above 7.0 alkalinity increases; below 7.0 acidity increases. Lemon juice and vinegar are mildly acidic, with a pH between 2.0 and 3.0. The pH of the hair and skin is around 5.0, slightly acidic.

Most good, natural skin cleansers, hair conditioners, and moisturizers have a pH between 3.5 and 5.5, so as not to irritate the skin. Natural ingredients, with their own natural pH, make the best cosmetics for your skin.

BRITTLE, SPLIT NAILS

The medical term for this problem (yes, there is a medical term) is *onychorrhexis,* splitting and brittleness of the nails. The exact causes of this condition are not known. When hands are frequently in hot water and in contact with harsh soaps, detergents, or other irritating substances, nails take the punishment. Frequent use of polish remover, which dries out the nail bed, is another common culprit.

Here's the explanation. When hands are immersed in water, the nail cells swell. Then when the nails dry, the cells shrink. With repeated swelling and shrinking, the nail will eventually split. Contrary to current opinion, the problem is not due to lack of protein, gelatin, calcium, or vitamins. There is not much calcium in the nail; its hardness is due to its special protein bonds. Extra protein or gelatin in the diet will not make our nails harder.

The best way to prevent fingernails from splitting is to keep your hands away from hot water, drying soaps, and detergents. Apply nail oil or cream often. Wear waterproof gloves for wet tasks. Cotton-lined gloves or a separate pair of cotton gloves inside rubber or vinyl gloves may offer the most protection. There are hypoallergenic gloves available now for those sensitive to latex, made from a material called nitrile™ that resists bleach and household solvents. (See page 251 for glove resources.) If these methods fail, what follows are some easy remedies to help brittle nails.

Salad hands. Mediterranean chefs use this remedy every time they make a salad. They rub the olive or avocado oil from the dressing into their nails and cuticles. Massaging the cuticle area increases circulation and encourages new nail growth. The oil seals in the moisture that is depleted when hands are in and out of water.

Did you know that because the nail is so porous, it gives off moisture a hundred times as fast as the skin?

Thuja. A homeopathic remedy for brittle nails is Thuja 6x. You should be able to obtain this treatment in stores selling medicinal herbs or from a homeopathic specialist.

Thuja 6x is made from the fresh, green twigs of the American arborvitae or Eastern white cedar. These branches contain thujone, a volatile oil that is said to affect the concentration of salt, water, and electrolytes in the body, as well as other wax, resin, and gelatinous ingredients. It encourages moisturization and helps prevent and heal brittle or split nails. Thuja is best in a homeopathic, diluted dose because it can be toxic when taken at full strength and in excess.

Caution: Pregnant women and people with irritant, dry coughs should not take thuja.

WHAT IS HOMEOPATHY?

The practice of homeopathy is centered on the belief *similia similibus curentur*, meaning "like cures like." Homeopathic practitioners use herbs, minerals, and animal extracts for their medicines. Homeopathic treatments involve the administration of minute diluted doses. For instance, if you were bitten by a snake, a homeopathic remedy might be a very dilute extract of snake venom.

A homeopathic remedy is first prepared in a solution as the "mother tincture." A small quantity is then diluted to one tenth (by the addition of nine parts alcohol or water) and shaken vigorously. A small quantity of this preparation is then diluted again to one tenth and shaken. This process is repeated again and again, producing weaker and weaker solutions identified as 3X (diluted three times), 6X (diluted six times), 30X (diluted thirty times), and so on, according to the number of dilutions.

HENNA NAIL PASTE

Henna has wonderful conditioning and nail-strengthening properties. This is a fun, natural nail treatment to do with children or on your own.

½ cup (125 ml) boiled water

½ teaspoon (2.5 ml) uncolored, neutral henna powder

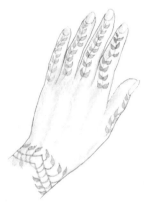

Mehndi henna design

To make:

1. Add the henna to the warm, boiled water and mix well, using a non-metal stirring spoon.

2. Make a paste of the mixture and place it in a small jar with a screw-top lid.

To use:

1. Using a chopstick, glob the henna paste on each of your clean, dry nails. Even though the henna is neutral, the color will be a soft green. This green will not remain on your nails, and it will not stain.

2. Let the henna paste dry on your nails and cuticles for 10 minutes. You will feel a pleasant "drawing" sensation.

3. Afterward, rinse your fingers, towel dry, and gently buff the nails.

4. You can use neutral henna once or twice a week for nail conditioning. Remember to stir the henna mixture each time.

MEHNDI: BODY ART WITH HENNA

Mehndi is the 5000 year-old traditional art of adorning the fingers, hands, forearms, toes, and shins with a non-permanent dye paste made from the leaves of the henna plant. Hand and body henna designs vary from large floral patterns in Arab countries to fine, lacy paisleys in India to bold geometric patterns in Africa. Henna designs will usually last for 4 to 6 weeks.

Painting with henna is more than a decorative art. In some countries people believe it to have healing properties, and it is used in place of gloves; in others, there is a mystical, protective connotation allied with its use, especially in marriage rituals.

SOOTHING NAIL AND CUTICLE OIL

Treat yourself to a warm, relaxing nail oil bath at least twice a week. Almond oil is a good base moisturizer for brittle or split nails. You can add the essential oils of sage, chamomile, lavender, or vanilla-like benzoin as helpful agents against any fungal infections or bacteria that might be hiding around the cuticles and under the nails. These oils also add a bit of aromatherapy to enhance your mood.

4 tablespoons (60 ml) pure sweet almond oil
20–25 drops of your choice of essential oil of sage, chamomile, lavender, or benzoin
1 vitamin E capsule (400 IU)

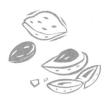

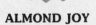

ALMOND JOY

Eat 6 raw almonds every day to relieve splitting of the fingernails. Linoleic acid, an essential fatty acid (EFA), is one of the important components of almonds. Among other benefits, EFAs help lubricate the body's cells.

To make:

1. Pour the almond oil into a small bottle and add the essential oil of your choice.

2. Pierce a vitamin E capsule and squeeze it into the mixture. Shake thoroughly.

3. Label the bottle with the contents and the date you created the blend.

To use:

1. When you are ready to use the blended oil, warm the bottle by setting it in a bowl of hot water for a few minutes.

2. Soak your nails in the blended oil for 10 minutes.

3. Sleep with cotton gloves on or wrap the hands in plastic wrap covered with a towel for at least 30 minutes for extra benefit.

For a massage: Give yourself or someone you look after a nail and hand massage before bedtime. Rub a few drops of the oil into the nails, cuticles, and skin. At the end of the massage, have the recipient rub his/her hands together, breathe deeply, and rest. The massage is relaxing and at the same time will stimulate circulation in the hands.

Caution: Essential oil of lavender is not recommended for those in the first trimester of pregnancy or who have very low blood pressure.

HORSETAIL NAIL BATH

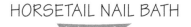

With a high content of silicic acid (5 to 8%), horsetail is a good astringent, antiseptic, and tissue and nail strengthener. On the days you are not using cuticle and nail oils, bathe your fingernails in this decoction of horsetail. Try this regimen over several months: one week of nail oil treatments alternating with one week of horsetail nail baths.

1 ounce (30 g) fresh horsetail in 1-inch (2.5 cm) pieces, sliced and bruised (or use the dried herb, cut and sifted)

Cold spring water to cover, about 1 pint (½ liter)

3 teaspoons (15 ml) sugar (helps to extract the silicon from the herb)

To make:

1. In a small pot with lid, cover the horsetail with water, add the sugar, and simmer for 30 minutes.

2. Let the decoction cool to a comfortable temperature.

To use:

Soak fingernails for 10 minutes.

HORSETAIL TEA FOR BRITTLE NAILS

When you want to attack the problem from both the inside and the outside, drink horsetail tea and use the Horsetail Nail Bath (above).

This is the way Jim Duke, author of *The Green Pharmacy,* prepares the brew.

2 teaspoons (10 ml) dried stems of horsetail herb

2 cups (500 ml) water

2 teaspoons (10 ml) sugar (helps to extract the silicon from the herb)

To make:

1. Put the horsetail in a stainless pot.

2. Cover with water and add the sugar. Bring to a boil and simmer for 3 hours.

3. Strain the liquid.

To use:

Drink 2 cups of the tea a day. You can double the amount of the recipe and store in the refrigerator; however, herbal water infusions and decoctions are best when fresh and should be used within one week.

BURDOCK SEED NAIL AND CUTICLE CONDITIONER

This recipe for an infused burdock seed oil is shared by Matthias Reisen of Healing Spirits Herb Farm in Avoca, New York. If you like going for extended walks and want to try your hand at wildcrafting (finding your own naturally grown herbs), start at the top. If you use purchased burdock seeds, skip ahead to the "To make:" section on the next page.

Burdock's effects on the skin have been valued from China to Chile, from Canada to Russia. The plant contains inulin, an essential oil, B-vitamins, and fatty acids. The seeds have a demulcent nature and help to restore smoothness to the skin and nails. Burdock is also an alterative and is suggested for treating chronic skin diseases.

Burdock seeds
Cold-pressed olive oil
Liquid contents of a 400 IU
    vitamin E capsule
    (optional)

To keep nails and cuticles in top form, some fashion models save empty, clean nail polish bottles and fill them with a light vegetable oil. They then brush this oil on their nails and cuticles several times during the day.

Wildcrafting and harvesting burdock:
If you've decided to collect your own *Arctium lappa* burrs, wear heavy-duty rubber gloves — these guys are clingers! Take a field guide to properly identify the plant.
1. Run your gloved hand up the stock and remove only the marble-size burrs. Put the burrs in a heavy-weight paper shopping bag or a woven plastic feed sack.
2. Wearing thick-soled shoes or boots, place the bag on a concrete floor or other hard surface. "Stomp" or crush the plant material, stepping heavily or jumping (you can also use a large mallet). This process is fun when you want to get rid of your aggressions (and have plenty of time). The seeds will come loose.
3. Shake the contents of the bag onto a metal ⅛" mesh screen, resting on a bucket filled with cold water.
4. Sift the tiny seeds into the bucket. The seeds will fall to the bottom. Discard the floating material and strain the water with a fine sieve to catch the seeds.
5. Place the wet seeds on a screen to dry for about 48 hours.

To make:

1. Grind the seeds once they are dry. (You may have the most success using a Japanese ceramic mortar, or *saribachi,* with a wooden pestle, or *suri kogi,* or using a stone mortar and pestle — see "Resources" on page 247 for suppliers.)

2. Put the ground seeds into a mason jar. Fill the jar with enough olive oil to cover the seeds with about an inch to spare.

3. Lightly screw on the lid (not tight) or cover the jar with a double fold of cheesecloth secured with a rubber band. Label the jar with contents and date, and then place the covered jar in a paper bag and set in a sunny window for two weeks.

4. Strain well twice, using a metal strainer lined with cheese-cloth or an unbleached paper coffee filter, to remove all bits of plant material.

5. Simply decant (pour off) the oil into dark-colored bottles, taking care not to allow any sediment to enter your new bottles.

6. If you wish, add a few drops of vitamin E oil as a preservative.

7. Cork or screw on a lid. Label the new bottles with the name of the herb and the date the oil was prepared.

To use:

Rub the oil into your cuticles and fingernails. Burdock seed oil is also good for dry scaly skin, cradle cap, eczema, and psoriasis.

WILDCRAFTING TIPS

♦ Be familiar with, or bring someone who is familiar with, the terrain. Do not harvest plants that may have been sprayed with toxic pesticides.

♦ Do not harvest plants that are near busy highways.

♦ Bring field guides to help you identify plants. Sometimes the variations within plant species are subtle. Part of the fun of learning about herbs and plants is becoming aware of the amazing adaptations that have occurred to ensure the plant's survival. (See page 250 for field guide suggestions.)

♦ Do not overharvest plant populations; pick sparingly, and leave plenty of each species in its natural habitat to sustain its population.

♦ Be aware of what plants and herbs are endangered and are struggling for sur-vival in the wild; in these cases, you may wish not to wildcraft but to purchase the plant or herb, and to verify with the supplier that the plant was obtained in a responsible manner.

NAIL FUNGUS

How does a fungus produce an infection? Nail fungi invade the superficial layers of the skin and in a few days germinate their spores along the edge of fingernails or toenails. A mass of fungal filaments grows into the nails. Fungi love to eat protein or keratin. Our nails become the "fertilizer" for these skin fungi, and our sweat glands provide the moisture to irrigate the crop.

Not everyone who comes in contact with fungi becomes infected. General health and nutrition play a role, as well as good hygiene practices. Scratching fungal infections on other places on your body such as your scalp or beard, or ringworm on your chest, or scratching pets with a skin condition can spread the problem to your fingernails.

The first step in treating a nail fungal infection is to have it diagnosed correctly. Once you know what you're dealing with, you can take the appropriate steps to treat it.

Tinea Fungal Infections

Fungal infections of the nails (*Tinea unguium*) will begin at the ends of the nails and then spread to occupy the entire nail bed. Over time the nail degenerates, becoming thickened, crumbly, white, or yellow. It can be painful, but is most often only unsightly. Those who tend to pick up athlete's foot may also be prone to develop *Tinea* infections on their fingernails. (Why is it that when we read about or write about things like this, we develop an incredible urge to scratch?)

To fight a *Tinea* fungal infection of the nail:

◆ First, have it diagnosed correctly.
◆ Add fresh garlic to your diet (5 cloves a day).
◆ Take tincture of echinacea daily; this herbal remedy helps the body rid itself of microbial infections.
◆ Keep your nails short and dry.
◆ Wear gloves for wet tasks.
◆ Clean under and around your nails with non-distilled witch hazel extract.
◆ Apply the Nail-Biters' Aloe Vera Ointment on the affected area (see page 58).
◆ Try several herbal, antifungal remedies individually until you find the one that works for you (see page 74).

Candida nail infections

Candida are a specific genus of yeastlike fungi. A *Candida* nail infection may look like a *Tinea* infection, but it may also have a creamy discharge. This kind of infection seems to attack those who frequently have their hands in soapy water without gloves. Generally, these nail infections are slow in healing but will respond to some form of antifungal cream or treatment.

The yeast species in food has nothing to do with the *Candida* that infect the skin. Changing to a yeast-free diet will not help cure a *Candida* infection of the nails.

To fight a *Candida* infection of the nail:

◆ Keep your nails short.
◆ Take B vitamins. Add wheat germ and yogurt with active cultures to your diet.
◆ Keep your hands out of water (what a great excuse to get the family to help out here!) or wear protective gloves.
◆ Use your hair dryer to blow warm air under the edge of the nails a couple of times a day to keep them dry.

Herbal Antifungal Remedies

Following are three herbal antifungal remedies in three types of delivery systems: a wash or soak, an essential oil, and a glycerin tincture. If you have a stubborn fungal infection of your fingernails, try each one of these recipes individually to see which works best for you. Tea tree oil may be the easiest to find, so start there. Improvement happens slowly with fungal infections; even prescription medications can take six months to a year to work.

RED CEDAR GLYCERIN TINCTURE

The red cedar, named for its cinnamon red bark that becomes gray-brown over time, is native to northwest America. Red cedar leaves have strong antifungal, antibacterial, and immunostimulant properties.

1 part red cedar leaves, crushed

2 parts glycerin mixture (50% glycerin, 40% water, 10% ethyl alcohol or vodka)

To make:

1. Put the crushed *Thuja plicata* leaves in a jar and cover with the appropriate amounts of glycerin, water, and alcohol.

2. Seal the jar, label, and store in a cool place for two weeks. Give the jar a turn every day, if possible.

3. After two weeks, strain twice through cheesecloth, pressing the liquid from the leaves.

4. Pour the strained liquid into clean, dark glass bottles. Seal and label.

To use:

Apply the tincture two to three times a day, with consistency, on the cuticle and under the free edge of the nail. You should begin to see some improvement at the end of one week.

Caution: Red cedar is not suggested for use during pregnancy or by those with kidney weakness.

MYRRH WASH OR SOAK

Myrrh, a bushy shrub native to Somalia and Saudi Arabia, has been prized for centuries for its fragrance and usefulness in cleansing and healing wounds. It is also considered an immune stimulant and an antifungal. You may even notice myrrh today as an astringent ingredient in mouthwashes and gargles for sore throat and mouth ulcers.

10 drops essential oil of myrrh or 2 teaspoons (10 ml) tincture of myrrh (see recipe below)

5 tablespoons (75 ml) comfortably warm spring water

To make:
Add the essential oil or tincture of myrrh to the warm water and stir well.
To use:
Use as a soak or a wash around and under the nails.
For stubborn infections: Take a tincture of myrrh (see recipe below) internally, 20 drops (1 ml) well diluted in half a glass of liquid, such as apple juice, three times a day with meals. (Myrrh is not noted for its pleasant taste.) Or take one 200 mg capsule three times a day.
Caution: If you are pregnant, avoid the use of myrrh, as it is also considered a uterine stimulant.

TINCTURE OF MYRRH

It is easy and inexpensive to make your own myrrh extract.

¼ cup (60 ml) crushed myrrh resin (available at most herb shops or wherever bulk herbs are sold)

¼ cup (60 ml) distilled water

¼ cup (60 ml) 190-proof grain alcohol

To make:
1. Combine the ingredients in a clean 6–8 ounce jar with a screw-top lid. Seal and label.
2. Steep for 3 to 4 weeks in a cool, dark place, turning daily.
3. Strain and rebottle in dark glass containers.

TEA TREE OIL DIRECT

The oil of tea tree is a broad-spectrum fungicide as well as an antibacterial and antiviral agent. It is also a soothing topical anesthetic. The clear, light, lemon-colored oil is best when packaged in amber or opaque containers to prevent chemical breakdown by light.

Essential oil of tea tree
Cotton swabs

To use:

1. For fungal infections of the nail, paint tea tree essential oil on clean, dry nails.

2. Use a cotton swab to dab the oil directly on the cuticle and under the free edge of the nail three times daily. Or massage the oil into the nail bed twice daily.

Caution: Some people are sensitive to tea tree oil. Try a patch test first on a small spot of non-infected skin. If your skin is reactive to full-strength tea tree oil, wash the area with soap and water. Then try cutting the strength of the essential oil by putting about 2 tablespoons of almond oil in a small glass bottle with 10 drops of tea tree oil. Shake well and paint around nails. Do not use tea tree oil near your eyes.

THE VERSATILE TEA TREE

The Australian aboriginal people have made use of the *Melaleuca* tree for at least a thousand years. They prepare a tea from the leaves, and make a leaf poultice remedy to apply directly to wounds. Following their example, during World War II Australian troops carried essential oil of tea tree in their first-aid kits as a powerful antiseptic, fungicide, and analgesic for cuts, abrasions, minor burns, toothaches, warts, and cold sores. Thursday Plantation was the first Australian company to commercialize the planting and growing of *Melaleuca* trees in New South Wales.

ASTRAGALUS ON THE MENU

When you have a nail fungus or infection, you may want to build up your general state of health. One of the easy things you can do is add astragalus to your diet. First, you have to learn how to pronounce it (uh-strag'-uh-lis), with the emphasis on the second syllable.

What it is: Astragalus is an herb from Chinese medicine whose root has been used since ancient times to stimulate the body's immune responsiveness. Recent studies indicate that astragalus causes specific components of the immune system, such as macrophages and T-suppressor cells, to become more active.

Where to obtain: You should be able to find these sticks (they look like doctor's tongue depressors) in Chinese markets. The Chinese word for astragalus is *Huang-qi*. (Write this name down before you go shopping. Otherwise, it may be very difficult to locate. I know.) You can find astragalus in small (3–4") or large (7–10") sticks.

How to add it to your diet: I prepare homemade chicken soup and while it's simmering, I drop in the dried root sticks along with the rest of my ingredients. For two gallons of soup stock, you could start with 4 to 6 small or 3 to 4 large dried root pieces. It won't change the flavor of your soup but it will work to enhance immune function, promote tissue regeneration, and improve circulation. Not bad for a simple root! You can also try preparing it as a tea, using 1 small stick (bruised) for each cup of water and drinking up to 3 cups daily.

CHAPTER 6
The Best Manicure

The activity of the hand runs through the whole history
of man and the life history of the individual.
— Geza Revesz
The Human Hand: A Psychological Study

The history of manicuring nails can be traced back four thousand years to southern Babylon, where noblemen used solid gold implements to manicure their fingernails and toenails. It was common for military commanders in ancient Rome and Egypt to have their nails painted to match their lips before leaving for battle. In Egypt, highborn men and women used henna to stain their nails — the deeper the red, the more important the person. Today, nail polish for men is having a resurgence in popularity. It's being marketed as stylish, fun, and sexy. Colors are olive, khaki, and black. You may be skeptical now, but just think, there was doubt when earrings for men were reintroduced. And now they are dangling from many an ear.

FINGERNAIL POLISH

Coloring the nails goes back to the Ptolemaic period of ancient Egypt around 30 B.C.E., when the fingertips were dipped in orange henna.

It is believed that fingernail polish was invented by the Chinese about five thousand years ago. Royal Chinese colors for nails were red and black gloss. At that time, long nails were a sign that one had the means to be idle and therefore symbolized wealth. People took extreme care to protect each long nail; the fingertips were encased in a gold or silver sheath lined with soft material.

The History of
Nail Polish Ingredients

During the Ming Dynasty, nail polish was made of beeswax, egg whites, gelatin, vegetable dyes, and gum arabic collected from the bark of the wild acacia tree.

Jumping ahead to the twentieth century, here is an American recipe from 1910 for nail varnish. In this period of U.S. history, it was considered vulgar or tawdry to have painted nails. Tints were massaged into the fingernails, and varnish, applied with a camel's-hair brush, had a life span of only one day.

1910 NAIL VARNISH

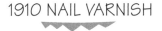

This recipe comes from *Beauty Culture,* a 1910 publication by William A. Woodbury.

1 tablespoon (15 ml) tincture of benzoin (available at most pharmacies)

1 tablespoon (15 ml) 100-proof grain alcohol

To make and use:

"Mix and paint upon the nail with a fine camel-hair pencil, after the second polishing, allow to dry on. The resulting light gloss will remain on for at least a day."

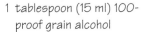

THE BIRTH OF NAIL POLISH

You can thank Henry Ford and his automobiles for the development of nail polish. After World War I, there was a large supply of leftover nitrocellulose, which had been used for military explosives. By trial and error, a brave soul experimenting with the material discovered that boiling the nitrocellulose causes it to become soluble in organic solvents. When these solvents evaporate, the resulting material is a glossy, hard lacquer.

Around 1920, the automobile industry became interested in developing this unique lacquer process for painting new, assembly-line cars. Nitrocellulose lacquer was the paint of choice for Fords. Not long afterward, the beauty industry refined the lacquer formula by adding softening resins as the basis for nail polish.

Ingredients in Today's Nail Products

Today, the basic ingredient in nail lacquer is still nitrocellulose, in a solvent that evaporates easily. Most nail polishes are chemically identical. Plasticizers, resins, and color give the polish gloss, depth, and staying power. The manufacture of nail polishes requires attention to detail. The factory must be in a temperature-controlled, explosion-proof facility equipped with generators in case of power failure — the high vapor pressure of the substances used in nail polish and lacquers can lead to explosions.

Nail polishes make the existing nail plate harder but, to the best of our knowledge, do not affect the nail matrix, the source of new nails.

There are two ingredients — toluene and formaldehyde — found in most nail polishes today that can cause reactions in particularly sensitive individuals. If you think you needed to read labels only in the supermarket, think again. If you find yourself having a reaction to either of these two chemicals, you should abstain from using nail polishes that include these chemicals in their ingredients list.

Toluene. Manufactured from petroleum by-products, toluene is one ingredient in nail polishes that can cause contact dermatitis. Many of the major cosmetic firms produce a nail enamel with a toluenesulfonamide, formaldehyde resin.

ALLERGY EVIDENCE

Allergic reactions to nail polish may surface first on your eyelids. If after applying a new nail polish your eyelids become red and swollen, this is your clue. Because eyelid skin is so delicate, it is particularly susceptible to contact dermatitis. (This means your nails or hands have rubbed your eyes.)

EAST BATON ROUGE PARISH LIBRARY
MAIN LIBRARY
Expiry date: 29 Jan 2022

Borrowed on: 04/17/2021 10:28 Till

1) Natural hand care : herbal
   treatments and simple techniques for
   healthy hands and nails
   Due date: 05/08/2021
   No : 31059019580329

Total on loan : 2

To renew items call 225-231-3740
or visit www.ebrpl.com
04/17/2021 - 10:28

Formaldehyde. Commonly used in nail hardeners, formaldehyde is a chemical preservative that can cause skin irritation and allergic reactions. The first clue to a formaldehyde sensitivity may be a rash around the cuticles. However, dermatologists report that formaldehyde reactions can include anything from dry or discolored nails to bleeding under, or loss of, a nail.

Continuing to use products with formaldehyde after developing a sensitivity may lead to problems with the nails separating from the nail bed. If you are reactive to this preservative, look for polishes labeled "formaldehyde-free" or be careful that the polish does not touch the skin.

NATURAL HOME MANICURE

Taking care of your hard-working nails can be a relaxing, pleasant, experience. Plan now to treat yourself to a scheduled home manicure every two weeks, and allow time for between-manicure touch-ups and nail maintenance as needed. (However, if a do-it-yourself manicure is not for you, you might still want to read through the following step-by-step instructions — they will help you decide the extent of a manicure you may want from a salon, as well as evaluate their techniques.) When done with a little care, a manicure will offer protection for your nails by eliminating rough edges, coating the nail surface, and helping to improve your self image.

Manicures were first introduced in the United States in barbershops. The original barber chair was built with a hollow in each armrest with bowls for hand-soaking. During a routine haircut and shave, customers primed their nails for manicures.

Put on your favorite music. Cut some flowers from the garden or buy a bouquet. Take a lazy bath and set the mood for feeling good.

Before you begin your manicure, take a good look at your nails and hands. Now is the time to plan your strategy for maintaining healthy, strong, well-groomed nails. Are your nails dry? Do they have lines or ridges? Are the nails peeling in layers? Are they soft or brittle? In what shape are your cuticles? Are you a nail-biter and do you have hangnails? Have you been eating right and getting some exercise and enough sleep? If you don't take care of yourself, no one else will. Don't be overwhelmed. Learning to walk begins with the first step.

TOOLS FOR THE PERFECT HOME MANICURE

Good, focused work light

Hand towel: For drying your hands, and to place under your hand as you apply polish to your fingernails

100% cotton squares or balls: Useful for removing nail polish; cotton is very absorbent and does not leave behind bits of fiber

Polish remover without acetone: To remove any nail polish before manicure begins; try to find one without acetone, as it is damaging to the nail (see Step 1 to the right)

Finger bowl: For soaking fingernails

Warm water: To clean nails and soften cuticles so they can be gently pushed back, if necessary

Soft nail brush: To clean under and over your fingernails

New flexible nonmetal nail file: To lightly shape and smooth nail edges (should be new or sanitizable to prevent the spread of germs)

Natural nail oil or moisturizer: Nails have to be moisturized, just like skin

Orange stick: For gently pushing back the cuticle (was traditionally made of orange wood, although today you may find it made of flexible plastic)

Chamois-covered nail buffer (optional): Used to rub gently over bare nails, bringing out their natural shine

Nail powder (optional): To encourage a shine while buffing

Clear base coat: To provide a foundation for the nail polish

Clear or tinted nail polish: The main coat of polish (a clear polish will usually last longer without showing chips or peels)

Top coat: A protective, durable coating for the polish (may contain sunscreen)

Hand lotion: To promote supple skin by hydrating and moisturizing

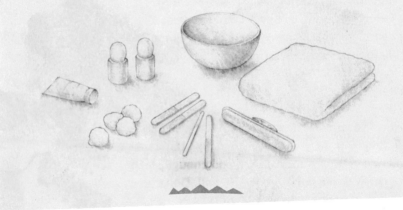

Step 1: Remove any polish from your nails

Partially saturate a cotton pad with the remover and work quickly to take up the old enamel. Start with the thumb. Use a cotton pad or swab to whisk off the polish with a rocking motion from the base of the nail to the tip. Do not smear the old polish into the cuticle or the surrounding tissues. Use this product sparingly and minimize skin contact. Never buy — and never be talked into using — a polish remover system that requires you to stick your entire finger into the jar of solution.

Polish removers are just not good for the nails. Avoid those containing acetone or chemical relatives of acetone, even if they say they have conditioners. This solvent degreases the nails, taking the oil out of them so that they cannot retain moisture. In addition, acetone and the alcohol in polish removers damage the surface of the nail, affect the nail's natural luster, and weaken and thin the nail plate. If you must use an acetone-based remover, dilute it with about 6 drops of olive or castor oil.

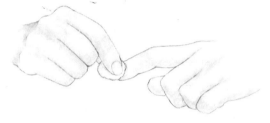

Step 2: Rinse

Rinse your fingernails in warm water immediately after using polish remover. Then scrub nails gently with a soft-bristle brush. Towel dry. If you apply moisturizer to your nails and hands while they are still a bit damp, it helps seal in the moisture.

If you've done this the night before the manicure, wear cotton gloves to bed for an extra skin treatment.

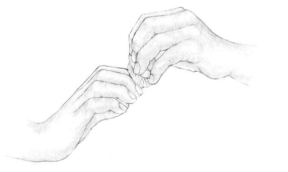

Step 3: File

Filing is necessary to shape and buff away any imperfections. File fingernails only when they are dry and free of cream.

When shaping nails, file from one edge of the nail to the center, and then from the other edge back to the center. Never file in the corners. Use long, smooth strokes and try not to saw the nail. Filing nails in the direction they grow prevents splitting.

For an easy filing position, make a fist and then uncurl your fingers slightly. File with your fingers facing you.

Keep your nails even and at a workable length for you. Softly square or oval tips are easier to maintain.

Step 4: Soak

Soak fingertips briefly in warm water after filing the nails. For a treat, try the Pineapple-Yogurt Nail Soak on page 85, or, if you suffer from infected or irritated nails, see the recipe for the Warm Flower Soak on page 61.

Stained nails: If your nails are stained, now is a good time to soak them for 10 minutes in a solution of 1 capful of hydrogen peroxide to 1 cup (250 ml) of warm water. You can repeat this practice once a week. After the soak, use a soft nail brush and scrub under the free edge of each nail with baking soda and water.

TO AVOID PEELING NAILS

◆ To maintain shape and an even surface, file your nails with a fine-grit file or round nail disk.

◆ Never peel away a torn, chipped, or split nail. Instead, use a scissors or nail clipper and a fine-grit file. This is especially important for you nail-biters.

◆ Don't allow your nails and cuticle area to become dry and rough. Try to apply a moisturizer or cuticle cream every time you wash your hands.

PINEAPPLE-YOGURT NAIL SOAK

This recipe is shared by Patricia Rivers-Sergienko, a natural nail care professional. Pineapple contains two helpful ingredients: bromelain, an enzyme that can reduce inflammation and pain, and alpha-hydroxy acids (AHAs), which peel off dead skin cells. Yogurt is very nourishing and a natural healer.

½ teaspoon (2.5 ml) apple cider vinegar
1 teaspoon (5 ml) olive oil
2 tablespoons (30 ml) pineapple juice, fresh or canned
2 tablespoons (30 ml) plain organic yogurt, regular or nonfat

To make:
1. Measure each ingredient and add to bowl.
2. Whip mixture with a fork until blended and creamy.

To use:
1. Dip fingers in the bowl and relax, allowing each hand to sit in the mixture for 5 minutes.
2. Massage both hands and fingers with the pineapple-yogurt mixture. Leave on skin for a few more minutes. Then rinse in warm water and pat dry. Use a fresh batch each time you do a manicure.

Step 5: Gently push back cuticles

Never cut your cuticles or push them back aggressively. The cuticle is the shield that protects the root of the nail — the matrix — from unfriendly bacteria and dirt. *Do not use cuticle removers.* Cuticle removers contain alkali and are among the harshest cosmetic products on a store's shelves. Regularly moisturizing the nail with an oil is a safer and more effective process for keeping the cuticles in good condition.

To gently push back the cuticle, use a soft, moist towel or an orange stick. Trim excess dead skin and hangnails with small, sharp scissors only when necessary. Never cut living skin.

Step 6: Clean under your nails

Avoid using a pointy or metal tool to clean under your nails. Instead, use a nail brush. Being too vigorous may create a space that allows fungi or bacteria to grow, so be gentle.

Step 7: Moisturize

Use a moisturizer on your cuticles, nails, and hands every time they have been in water. This is an ideal to work toward. The best store-bought skin moisturizer will contain phospholipids (natural emulsifiers and humectants), urea, and/or lactic acid. You can also try unrefined avocado oil or pure jojoba liquid. Or prepare a natural recipe such as Perfect Moisturizing Hand Cream (page 111) or Chatham Chap Cream (page 137).

Step 8: Massage

This is a good time to massage your hands. If you like, turn on some music that is soothing to your spirit. These strokes are adapted from those suggested by Michael Reed Gach, author of *Arthritis Relief at Your Fingertips*. Rub on a moisturizing cream, or mix 1 tablespoon (15 ml) of gently warmed avocado oil with 3 to 5 drops of your favorite pure essential oil and allow your hands to savor the experience.

Palm rub. Rub your palms together briskly to create some warmth, and then rub the backs of each hand.

Back of hands press. Clasp the fingers of both hands together with the palms facing. Squeeze the fingertips against the back of your hands. Hold for 5 to 10 seconds. Relax. Breathe deeply. Repeat.

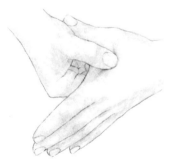

web pinch

Web pinch. The space between each of your fingers is the web. Pinch between the thumb and the index finger, hold for a moment, then rub. Repeat this process between each of the fingers on both hands. Eastern therapies hold that applying pressure on the finger's web sites (not the Internet!) helps to dispel headaches and move toxins from the body.

Finger circles. Use your opposite hand to gently stretch and make little circles with each finger and thumb. Reverse direction of finger rotation. Repeat on the other hand.

Wrist compress. Support the wrist of one hand with the palm, fingers, and thumb of the other and squeeze lightly for about five seconds. Next, create the motion of a washing machine by gently rotating back and forth the wrist being held in the grasp of the supporting hand, while gently moving the holding hand in the opposite direction. Give the other wrist the same gentle treatment.

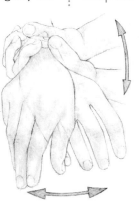

Forearm press. Knead the outer muscle of the forearm below the elbow. Push the tips of your four fingers sensitively into the skin, using the thumb as anchor, and work slowly up and down the arm, about three times, as if you were kneading bread dough. Repeat on the other arm.

Elbow rub. Take this opportunity to moisturize the elbow and forearm with your favorite cream or lotion by massaging with the fingertips of the opposite hand in circular movements from the elbow down to the wrist, then over the hand and fingers.

Arm and finger stretch. Interlace the fingers of both hands with the palms facing and then slowly turn the palms outward. Stretch your arms in front of you and give the fingers and arms an easy, relaxed stretch. Release and shake out your hands as if you were trying to dry your nails.

Step 9: Apply polish

If you are going to use nail polish, wet a corner of a soft cotton towel and wipe any remaining cream from the nails. Pat dry.

The best way to apply nail polish is in three coats: a clear base coat followed by the polish, and topped with a clear top coat to lock in the color.

Applying nail polish can be tricky for the inexperienced, so here are some tips to start you off:

- ◆ Allow the clear base coat to dry for 3 minutes before applying the polish; this will act as a foundation for the polish and help to prevent nail stains caused by colored nail polish.
- ◆ Do the thumb last; it can be a helpful tool for mopping up polish spills on the cuticles of your other fingers.

- Blend nail polish by rolling the bottle between your palms. (Shaking causes air bubbles.)
- When you are applying polish, work in a well-ventilated room so that you will not breathe in the vapors.
- Using a clear polish rather than a colored one has its advantages — it shows less wear and doesn't have to be changed as often.
- Apply polish to the underside of the free edge of the nail, and then from the base of the nail to its free edge.
- Apply nail polish in two thin coats. Use three strokes from base to tip. First polish up the center, then up each side. Let the first layer dry for 3 minutes and the second for 5 minutes.
- Avoid quick-dry polishes; they most likely contain acetone, which can parch your nails. A thicker, slower-drying polish will hold the moisture and give your nails more flexibility.
- Brush on a top coat to lock in the color and protect the polish.

Note: Long-term use of colored polishes may discolor the natural nail.

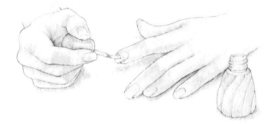

STAYING POWER

To increase the longevity of your nail polish application, before applying the first base coat, dip your unpolished fingernails into a mixture of white vinegar and warm water. Use this formula:

2 teaspoons (10 ml) white vinegar
1/2 cup (125 ml) warm water

Step 10: Buffing

If you decide you want an alternative to nail polish, try nail buffing. (It is not necessary to buff nails before applying polish.) Buffing will shine your nails, smooth away ridges, and improve circulation to the fingertips.

Use either a dry paste (see recipe for Tinted Nail Buffing Cream on page 90) or some light vegetable oil and a chamois-covered nail buffer.

For a natural gloss, buff the nails gently in one direction, with downward strokes from the base to the free edge of the nail. Raise the buffer after each stroke (otherwise you'll begin to feel a burning sensation). About 10 strokes lightly on each nail should be adequate.

Caution: Vigorous buffing, with heavy pressure, can cause ridges and thinning of the nails. If your nails are thin, limit buffing to once a month.

Caution for children: Do not buff children's nails — they have their own natural glow, and buffing can thin the nail's surface.

According to Beatrice Kaye, the original MGM movie studio manicurist, the rage in nail polish in 1924 was the "moon manicure." The free edge of the nail was point-shaped, and the polish was applied only to the center of the nail. The moon and the free edge of the fingernail were left uncovered.

TINTED NAIL BUFFING CREAM

Alkanet, an important dye plant, is also known as dyer's or Spanish bugloss. It is a lovely perennial with a purple-brown root native to the eastern Mediterranean. The name comes from the Spanish *alcanna,* derived from an earlier Arabic word for henna.

½ cup (125 ml) sweet
  almond oil
1 tablespoon (15 ml)
  alkanet root, powdered
¼ ounce (7.5 g) beeswax
Up to 30 drops of essen-
  tial oils of your choice
  (for extravagant pam-
  pering, try a combina-
  tion of otto of rose and
  violet)

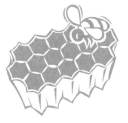

To make:

1. Pour the almond oil in a bottle or jar and add the powdered alkanet root. Stir together, and then seal, label, and refrigerate for two weeks. Gently shake the bottle daily.

2. After two weeks, the oil will be cranberry in color. Strain it through a coffee filter and bring to room temperature.

3. Melt the beeswax in a double boiler. Slowly stir in the alkanet oil. Remove from heat and add the essential oils of your choice.

4. Pour into cosmetic jars and label. Let sit overnight before using.

To use:

1. Spread a thin layer of the cream directly on the nails. Gently rub it in and leave undisturbed for a few minutes.

2. Buff with a nail buffer toward the free edge of the nail and lift the buffer after each stroke.

ARTIFICIAL NAILS

Artificial nails are not recommended and can lead to unnecessary nail and skin problems if not properly applied and maintained. However, if you choose to use them, know that there are at least two kinds of synthetic nails, each with their own advantages and drawbacks. My advice is, don't wear artificial nails for longer than three months at a time, if at all. Remove them for one month to give the natural fingernails a rest. Continue to take care of your fingernails during this time.

Preformed Synthetic Nails

A preformed synthetic nail is glued to the existing nail. The adhesive may cause irritation around the nail and later cause the real nail to separate from the nail bed. If you have any question about allergic reactions to the materials in artificial nails, have one test nail done and wait a few days to see if a reaction develops.

Note: Never use household glues for nail repairs. Use only products intended for nail care, and follow directions.

Acrylic Nails and Nail Wraps

An acrylic nail comes in liquid form. It is mixed with powder, which thickens and is molded around the natural nail. As the natural nail grows, you need more acrylic to fill in close to the nail bed. Acrylic nails can cause severe allergic reactions under and around the fingernails, and may even cause loss of nails.

Nail wraps and extensions repair natural breaks and lengthen fingernails with silk, fiberglass, or linen. The problem with nail wraps is that the surface of the nail must first be dehydrated so that resin or glue may be applied, and when it comes time to remove these wraps, chemical dissolving agents are used.

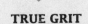

TRUE GRIT

The emery board was invented in 1910 by Flowery Manicure Products. It was a garnet abrasive on a wood center and a coarse 100 to 150 grit. Today, there are many choices of files. Here's the inside story so that you can make some informed decisions as to which ones to own.

Most files come in fine, medium, and coarse grit. The higher the grit number, the finer the abrasive, and the more gentle on natural fingernails.

Fine grit is the best for filing natural nails and for buffing artificial nails. For fragile fingernails, look for a #900 grit file.

Medium grit is okay for filing strong, natural nails, foot calluses, and synthetic nails.

Coarse grit is too rough for natural nails. It's about #80 grit and better for artificial surfaces.

Cushioned files have a layer of foam sandwiched between two filing surfaces. They are more flexible than basic files and the cushioning gives them weight and spring. There are two-sided file/buffers and three- or four-way file/buffers with different textures for smoothing the nail edge, removing ridges, and buffing.

Round nail disks offer the advantage of being able to buff the nail surface without scraping the important cuticle.

Emery boards, the old standby, are fine to take along in a handbag for quick repairs but a bit too coarse for the full manicure. They also lose their grit very quickly.

Metal files are really for artificial nails. The surface is too coarse and can leave jagged edges on your natural nails.

SALON MANICURE

When you need or want someone else to take care of your nails, a day spa or salon is where you'll head. Every now and then it's important to feel pampered. A professional touch can also enhance your self-image and sense of confidence.

Manicurists, nail technicians, and their salons are regulated by state and federal laws to protect customers from contracting infections or other problems as a result of their services. Each state has its own Board of Registration of Cosmetology that decides the regulations and oversees health procedures. These regulations help reduce customers' risks but every consumer needs to be his or her own best advocate. Every beauty establishment is required to have two licenses on prominent display: the state business license and the state board license. In addition, all nail technicians must display or have handy their manicurist licenses at their individual work stations.

Ask your nail tech if he or she is licensed and if the salon is licensed. If you don't see a license, inquire. Ask about the experience of your nail professional and whether he or she is staying current with refresher courses.

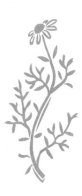

A DAY SPA'S MANICURE MENU

Some of the new day spas offer the client a menu of services that sound good enough to eat. Here's a sample of treats from one delicious-sounding spa:

Buff and Polish: Keep a refined look at all times — shape, buff, and polish of choice.
The French Manicure: A classic manicure, topped with a gentle pink polish and tipped white. Elegance at your fingertips.
Classic Manicure: A traditional manicure, complete with warm oil and fragranced salt soak, gentle hand and arm massage, nail shaping and cuticle care, followed by the polish shade of your choice.
Seaweed Aromatherapy Manicure: Surround your sense of smell with a seaweed aromatic essential oil bath and comforting clay mask followed by a Classic Manicure.
Spa Manicure: This invigorating hand and arm treatment includes exfoliating massage with dead sea salts and essential oils, followed by a Classic Manicure.
Soothing Paraffin Hand Treatment: Reward your deserving hands with a gentle massage and our special-blend glycolic moisturizer. Your hands are then submerged in a warm, nourishing vitamin E paraffin bath and wrapped in cozy terry mitts, leaving your skin velvety smooth.

Our implements are ultrasonically disinfected as hygiene is a primary concern. Complimentary professional jewelry cleaning completes your hand beautification.

Nail Salon Pointers

Here are some guidelines for choosing a health-conscious nail salon that observes hygienic manicure procedures and safe maintenance of equipment. These guidelines are based on statutory criteria and regulations from the Board of Registration of Cosmetology in Massachusetts.

◆ Is the facility neat and clean? Select a salon the way you would choose a restaurant: When you walk in, ask yourself, "Would I want to eat here?"

◆ Is there a strong smell of fumes? If there is, it's a sign that the place is poorly ventilated. Inhaling the fumes from nail products is not good for you or your nail tech.

◆ Is there a pre-service scrub? The nail technician should wash his or her hands thoroughly with hospital-grade antibacterial soap and hot water before and after each patron. Wash your hands, too!

◆ A fresh, clean towel must be used for each customer. Clean towels must be kept in a closed cabinet.

◆ Creams and other solid substances must be removed from containers with a clean spatula or tool. Cream containers should be kept closed when not in use.

◆ Manicure implements must be properly sterilized *after each use.* If you haven't brought your own manicure tools, be curious how the salon's tools are sterilized. Warts, infections, and blood-borne pathogens can be transmitted if the tools are not sterile. Preferred methods are autoclaving (heat sterilization), ultrasound cleaning, chemical sterilization with hospital-grade disinfectants, and bleach washes (see page 95). A heat-pressurized sterilizer offers the most secure protection. Sanitized instruments should be stored in an airtight container.

◆ No manicurist shall provide services to a person with a fungus infection of the nails.

SANITIZING BLEACH WASH

Whether you're sanitizing your own manicure equipment or inquiring into the sanitizing procedures of your nail salon, these are the proper guidelines for a sanitizing bleach wash. Remember, washing with bleach alone will not kill spores or hepatitis virus. In a nail salon, equipment should also undergo heat sterilization or ultrasound cleaning

½ cup (125 ml) bleach
1 quart (1 liter) water

To use:

1. Wash the implements first, then immerse them in the bleach, shake, and rinse. Repeat this procedure twice.

2. Dry the tools with a clean paper towel and place in a closed cabinet.

Note: For smaller or larger washes, increase or decrease the amounts of bleach and water proportionately, maintaining a 1 to 10 ratio.

SECRETS FOR NAIL FITNESS

◆ Try not to use your nails as tools. Fingernails are too special to be nature's screwdrivers.

◆ Always wear gloves while doing the dishes. Before putting on gloves, apply your favorite hand cream. The heat from the warm water will help your skin to absorb the cream. (This tip from Patricia Rivers-Sergienko.)

◆ To keep nails clean while doing dirty work, first scratch your nails over a bar of soap and then put on the appropriate gloves.

◆ It is much better to file your nails, but if you want to clip them, do so only when they are wet (after a shower or a bath).

◆ Clip baby's nails after a bath. Use blunt-end scissors and trim the nail in a curved edge following the natural shape. Press the tip of the finger down and out of the way as you cut. (See special baby nail scissors and kit by Tweezerman in "Resources.")

◆ Gelatin and calcium supplements will not strengthen or harden your fingernails. There is no substitute for eating fresh fruits, vegetables, and grains; drinking enough water every day; and getting basic exercise and proper rest.

Your Own Personal Manicure Tools

To reduce the chances of unwanted germs and possible infection, consider bringing your own manicure tools to the salon, such as a hand towel, scissors or nail clippers, a soaking bowl, a fine-grit file, an orange stick, a chamois buffer, and anything else you may need. Tools may seem an expensive luxury but they are much cheaper than the price of even one antibiotic.

I know a manicurist who keeps personalized tools for each of her clients in labeled sacks. It's a great idea!

Shaggy Dog Story

You may feel that I am going on beyond what is necessary to tell you about the importance of sanitary procedures, but a good salon will want to do these things for its staff as well as for you.

To make my point, here's a "shaggy dog" story I want to share. Several months ago I was walking through a mall when I passed a nail salon that advertised walk-in service, a price of only $10 for a plain manicure, and start-to-finish in 30 minutes. It was not my usual habit, but I opted for the manicure. During the process, the manicurist asked if I wanted her to cut my cuticles as they were hanging over my nails. I said, "okay" and she cut, and then my cuticle started to bleed. Somehow, I didn't have a good feeling about this. When I got home, I immediately put on some first-aid cream, but to no avail. The skin around the cuticle was red and swollen. It did not go away. After a month of trying herbal and other remedies, I went to see my physician, who prescribed an oral antibiotic. Still no change. Then I went to see a hand surgeon, who looked at the swelling on the knuckle and felt the clicking in the joint. He suggested a shot of cortisone — ouch! — and told me that the finger was becoming arthritic.

I am a lefty. As I write this, I am looking at the most important finger on my left hand, the index finger. I'm convinced it's ruined forever, and all because I was impulsive and not informed as to how to evaluate the safety of a nail salon. I didn't know how important it is to leave your cuticles alone. How did that salon clean its tools? Did the technician clean her tools between customers? A hard lesson learned. If I'm able to prevent even one of you from experiencing this problem, it will have been worth the telling.

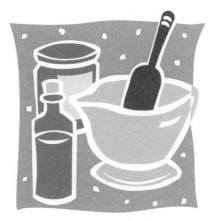

Skin Care for Your Hands: Everyday Protection and Simple Remedies

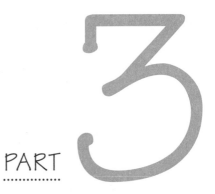

PART

3

CHAPTER 7
Basic Steps to Beautiful Hands

*Healing is simply attempting to do more of those things
that bring joy and fewer of those things that bring pain.*
— O. Carl Simonton, *The Healing Journey*

Our skin is the shield that protects the inner body from the stones and arrows of the outside environment. If you want a warranty from the manufacturer for long-term use, it's essential to find a natural routine that takes care of and maintains this protective equipment.

SUNBATHING IN THE NUDE

I knew that would get your attention! Nude sunbathing is what you do every time you venture out without covering your hands and arms with protective clothing or sunscreen. Depleting ozone layers dictate that you must protect the skin from the effects of ultraviolet radiation, both UVA and UVB — and if our ozone layer continues to be consumed, it will soon be UVC as well. Photoaging of the skin (rough, leathery texture, sagging skin, and brown-pigmented, freckle-like spots on the backs of the hands) is caused by undue exposure to sunlight.

Here's how. Long-term sun exposure degrades the skin's support network of collagen and elastin fibers and causes the skin to become less flexible. Research also points to other possible problems with excess sunbathing that include precancerous or cancerous growths due to changes in the body's DNA codes, and the possibility of a compromised immune response due to destruction of certain white blood cells (the helper T-cells). Each individual is different, and so is tolerance to sun exposure. Every one of us deserves some sunshine in our lives, but for beautiful, healthy skin, moderation is the key. If you're going to be outdoors for any length of time, wear sunscreen. It will protect your skin against sunburn and premature wrinkles. And don't forget to apply sunscreen to your hands.

GLOVES FOR EVERY REASON

Human skin comes wrapped and sealed with its own natural skin cream made of sebum, lecithin, cholesterol, and water. We do our best to break down this natural environmental barrier using hot water, detergents, solvents, polishes, and waxes that dehydrate the skin and remove its natural protective oils. Need an example? We have such a compulsion to keep things clean and shiny that it is difficult to keep our naked hands out of hot water. This behavior often results in "dishpan hands" and yeast infections around the nails. In solving this dilemma, it's gloves to the rescue. Whether you are washing, cleaning, or otherwise handling harsh materials, wear gloves to protect your hands against the elements.

Fabrics for gloves have come a long way from the days of metal chains, linen, and silk. Today gloves and mittens are made from every material you can think of, including canvas, cotton, nylon, terry cloth, wool, cowhide, deerskin, goatskin, latex, pigskin, polypropylene, rubber, suede, split leather, and vinyl.

Gloves are also available in every color of the rainbow and more. There are camouflage gloves for sportsmen; garden gloves with floral prints; water-repellent gloves with cotton-knit lining in colors coordinated to match any kitchen; and fluorescent, neon gloves with foam insulation and fleece lining ideal for shoveling snow while also making the occasional lost glove visible in a snowy yard.

IF THE GLOVE FITS, WEAR IT

There are varieties of gloves available today for every purpose you can imagine, and even for some you never imagined. In many cases, each glove is designed and manufactured to protect the hand against a particular environmental, chemical, or skin-destructive condition. On pages 102 and 103, you'll find a few examples of gloves for different tasks. For suppliers that carry these types of gloves, see page 251 of "Resources."

THROW DOWN THE GAUNTLET

Gloves have probably been worn since Adam left the cozy Garden of Eden. The earliest remnants of gloves have been found in Egypt, in the tomb of the pharaoh Tutankhamen, dating about 1350 B.C.E. In the Middle Ages, knights used gloves both as a challenge to combat and as a pledge of honor. Throwing a glove on the ground to be picked up by the person being challenged was the way a duel was arranged. In Scotland, "to bite a glove" was considered a pledge of vengeance that could be ended only by death.

At jousts during this age of chivalry, the glove was a love token a lady presented to her knight to be worn on his helmet during battle. Gloves in those days were handmade of linen, silk, velvet, or kid and were highly ornamented. Knights in armor protected their own hands with fingerless gloves, strengthened by chain mail or metal plates.

It wasn't until 1834 that gloves became available to regular folks not endowed with the riches of nobles, bishops, emperors, or queens. In that year, Xavier Jouvin, a glovemaker in Grenoble, France, invented the punch press, which simultaneously cut out six gloves and so spawned mass production. Not long afterward, in 1845, the invention of the sewing machine completely revolutionized glove making. Cotton and synthetic materials also helped to put gloves in the price range and reach of the general population.

Glove Tips for Gardening and Wet Work

Gloves are particularly useful for gardening and working in wet or cold conditions. They'll protect your hands from irritants such as fertilizers and pesticides and keep the skin from becoming raw and chapped. (Garden glove tips come courtesy of horticulturists Bruce Roberts and Suzanne Siegel of the Massachusetts Horticultural Society.)

- Always wear gloves when you have to do wet work.
- Cotton gloves do not provide adequate hand protection when working with plant pesticides or other chemicals. It's wiser to use lined, industrial-grade, rubber-type gloves for these applications. Recheck gloves for splits before each use and toss those that don't meet specs.
- Dark brown, cotton knit jersey gloves, available in various densities, are just right for working with tender plant material, especially for transplanting seedlings. You'll find them comfortable, durable, and washable.
- High-cuff leather gloves are what you need to protect your hands when pruning roses, shrubs, and trees.
- Choose gloves with a natural fiber lining to protect hands against possible allergic reactions.
- Make sure the gloves are long enough so that water or chemicals will not splash inside when you are engaged in messy work.
- Try not to wear gloves for wet work for more than one hour at a time.
- If you do have a skin condition such as eczema on your hands, be sure to turn your gloves inside out several times a week and wash them.
- Inspect gloves daily, prior to wearing, to ensure that there are no holes or tears to either the inside or the outside surface.
- Discard torn gloves.

Glove	Purpose/Description
Baker's mitts and potholders	Have an inner, protective barrier to shield against steam and grease; flame-retardant, with a wipe-clean surface
Curved fingers, contour palm gloves	Mimic the actual shape of the hands for longer wear and comfort
Disposable gloves	For food processing, restaurant use, dental and medical applications; sheer and stretchable
Driving gloves	For cushioning and durability, deerskin, pigskin, and cowhide; for the softest, most durable leather, try goatskin, with its own natural lanolin
Fingertip gloves	Fingertip-size for protection after finger surgery, handling small parts, or buffing and cleaning jewelry and electronics
Fishing gloves	Neoprene material with water-repellent seams; may come with waffle grip palm to keep the big ones from getting away
Fish preparation glove	Stainless-steel, to help you fillet just the fish and not your fingers; fits either hand
Garden gloves	To protect hands against irritants and abrasions from wet and dirty work; often made of leather, rubber, or canvas
Golf gloves	Promote better grip; protect against sun exposure and calluses; venting for long fingernails and oversize finger rings
Machine shop gloves	To protect the hands from oils, grease, acids, solvents, abrasion, cuts, and punctures; liquid-proof
Reflective gloves	For long-range night visibility to 350 feet; for law enforcement, fire personnel, joggers, bikers, walkers, construction workers
Ski gloves	To trap heat and block wind and cold; moisture-wicking fleece lining, with lofted air space to circulate warm, dry air; shaped to fit the natural curve of the hand

Glove	Purpose/Description
Skinlike gloves	For jobs that require dexterity, fine touch, and protection, and for those sensitive to latex
Sleep-in gloves	For comfort and breathability; medium-weight, cotton jersey
Warmer gloves	Microwavable, heat up against the cold
Welder's gloves	Heavy-duty, heat- and fire-resistant
Work or chore gloves	Protect against sharp edges and rough surfaces, heat, cold weather, repetitive tool abrasion, raw skin or pressure sores; look for durable leather padding on index finger, palm, and across knuckles; waterproof, high gauntlet, or security cuffs for added protection
Wrist-support gloves	Fingerless, lycra material

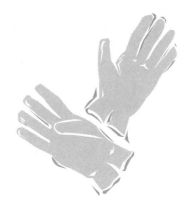

NATURAL HAND CLEANSERS
AND MOISTURIZERS

Washing your hands often is one of the best ways to stop the spread of germs and remove harmful atmospheric pollutants. Choose mild, natural ingredients for your hand cleansers, and apply barrier creams after cleansing to preserve the skin's moisture. This may surprise you, but pure water is one of the best ways to cleanse the skin. Water will remove soluble environmental pollutants such as compounds of sulfur and nitrogen, metal salts, and other chemicals, and with a neutral pH of 7.0, water accomplishes all this without disturbing the natural acid mantle of the skin.

Normal skin has a pH factor of 4.0 to 6.0. Tests show that skin with a normal pH of 4.0 rises to a pH of 7.0 one minute after washing with soap. If cider vinegar, which has a pH between 3.0 and 4.0, is applied to the skin after bathing, the pH factor will return to its normal range. However, the secret with skin-care products is to look for those that use natural ingredients. Avoid harsh, synthetic chemicals.

Natural and Herbal Hand Cleansers

Milk, sour milk, cream (used by Cleopatra, it is said), and buttermilk are all gentle skin cleansers. The next time you're in the kitchen, try washing with ¼ cup (60 ml) of fresh or sour milk, buttermilk, or cream instead of one of the liquid dish detergents. It is a surprisingly pleasant experience.

To remove greasy substances not removed by water or milk, try an exfoliant such as cornmeal or oatmeal. A heavy hand is not needed. The grainy texture releases both dirt and dead surface skin while stimulating the new skin cells below. Or try the Grainy Hands Soap Substitute recipe on page 105. (See chapter 8 for more recipes to care for bothered skin, such as the Oatmeal Hand Bath on page 147 or the Special Wash for Chapped Hands on page 135.)

GRAINY HANDS SOAP SUBSTITUTE

Make a batch to have "on hand."

1 cup (250 ml) cornmeal or oatmeal, finely ground

2 cups (500 ml) white kaolin clay, finely powdered

1/4 cup (60 ml) almonds, finely ground (leave just a bit of grittiness)

1/8 cup (30 ml) dried lavender blossoms, finely powdered

1/8 cup (30 ml) dried rose petals, finely powdered

A few drops of the essential oil of your choice (optional)

A pinch of dried kelp (optional)

A pinch of powdered vitamin C (optional)

Liquid contents of a 400 IU vitamin E capsule (optional)

To make:
Stir all ingredients together in a bowl and pour into a large jar. Store jar in a dry, cool location.

To use:
1. Mix 1 to 2 teaspoons (5–10 ml) of the cleansing grains with water.
2. Stir into a paste by rubbing your hands in a circular motion. Then work the grains up each individual finger and over the back of the hand.
3. Rinse with cool or lukewarm water. Pat dry.

Caution: This recipe may irritate bothered skin.

(Adapted from a recipe by master herbalist Rosemary Gladstar.)

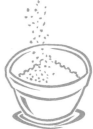

GRAINY HANDS SOAP SUBSTITUTE
FOR CHAPPED HANDS

This is a variation of the Grainy Hands recipe for people whose hands are raw or chapped. Make small batches on an as-needed basis.

1–2 teaspoons (5–10 ml) Grainy Hands Soap Substitute (see page 105)
1 scant teaspoon (5 ml) honey
Distilled rose water

To make:
Add honey to the Grainy Hands Soap Substitute and enough rose water to make a paste.

To use:
1. Stir into a paste by rubbing your hands in a circular motion. Then work the grains up each individual finger and over the back of the hand.

2. Rinse with cool or lukewarm water. Pat dry.

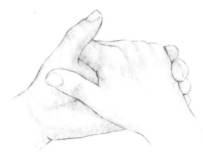

LEMONADE HANDS

This is a simple recipe that offers great results in improving the texture of your skin, shared with us by a lovely grandmother from Chile. Her hands belie her age and she confided that she has used this recipe every day for years. It smoothes the skin and acts as a mild exfoliant.

1 tablespoon (15 ml) granu-
    lated sugar
Fresh lemon juice to make
    a paste

To make:

1. Pour about 1 tablespoon of granulated sugar in the palm of your hand.

2. Squeeze enough juice from a fresh lemon wedge to make a paste.

To use:

1. Rub your hands together in a rotary motion, either clockwise or counterclockwise. At first, the sensation will be one of a gritty surface.

2. Continue rubbing. The heat of your hands will melt the sugar to become a candy glaze.

3. Work this glaze up and over each finger and over the back of each hand. Picture yourself as Lady Macbeth as she says, "Out out damned spot!" and really rub your hands.

4. Leave the glaze on your hands for 5 minutes.

5. Rinse with warm water. Pat your hands totally dry with a soft paper towel.

Skin Brushing

Popular in northern Europe, skin brushing with a dry loofah or soft, natural-bristle brush is an invigorating way to slough off dead skin and stimulate circulation. You can do it yourself or make it a mutual experience. To brush the skin of your hands, use a light touch and circling movements in a brisk, flicking, upward direction. Begin with brushing the fingers, then move up the hands to the arms, toward the heart. Choose the firmness of the brush according to your skin type. The more fragile your skin, the more gentle the brush. *Caution:* Do not practice skin brushing on areas affected by rashes, eczema, or psoriasis.

A natural sponge gourd *(Luffa cylindrica)* is generally a good choice for skin brushing. A tropical plant native to Asia and Africa, its fruit fibers remain after the fruit has decayed and are uncommonly resistant to molds even when they are continually kept wet.

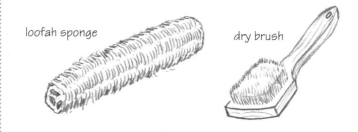

loofah sponge

dry brush

BRUSH FOR BETTER CIRCULATION

Physiologist Bernell Baldwin, Ph.D., theorizes that regular daily skin brushing will tone the vasomotor, or blood vessel, system of the body, making it more efficient. The conditioned vasomotor system may be better able to respond to extremes in temperature for improved blood circulation and delivery of oxygen to the cells. Those with Raynaud's phenomenon may want to try skin brushing as a therapy. (For more on this topic, see page 206.)

Natural and Herbal Hand Creams

If you want smoother, more pliable skin, get in the habit of using protective hand and nail creams. These creams help the skin retain moisture by adding to the natural, water-resistant (lipid) barrier between you and the environment. Soaps and detergents constantly erode this barrier. When applied to slightly damp skin, emollient creams, lotions, and ointments slow evaporation and hold on to vital moisture.

Which moisturizers are the best? The choice is yours. You might decide that at work you want a hand emollient that dries quickly and has no fragrance, has an oil-in-water (O/W) base, and is a lotion formula. At home you may use a water-in-oil (W/O) base, a cream formula, and one that you can wear all night with cotton gloves.

FROM THE FARM

Hand salves and creams have probably been around since the first peoples discovered bear grease. Many nineteenth-century hand products from the agricultural farm communities came with names like Absorbine Veterinary Liniment, Bag Balm, Corn Huskers Lotion, Thayer's Medicated Superhazel, and White Cloverine Salve. Farmers began to try these products, on the theory that "what's good for the horse is good for his owner."

One product, B and O'R Hand Lotion, conceived and produced by Vermont pharmacists Beauchamp and O'Rourke, was devised to cope with the industrial revolution. It was intended to protect ironworkers' hands from the temperature extremes of blast furnaces and the bitter Vermont cold. Witch hazel, camphor, soap liniment, glycerin, bay rum, rose water, and mutton tallow are some of the ingredients. It is still manufactured and sold today. (See "Resources" for the address of the Vermont Country Store Apothecary.)

KITCHEN CABINET HAND LOTION

2 teaspoons (10 ml) cod-liver oil

2 tablespoons (30 ml) castor oil

2 soy lecithin capsules, pierced and squeezed

1 natural vitamin E capsule, pierced and squeezed

1 tablespoon (15 ml) unflavored gelatin

1/4 cup (60 ml) cold water

3/4 cup (180 ml) boiling water

(Adapted from a recipe by Charles Dickson and Ariel Mars.)

To make:

1. In a blender, combine the cod-liver oil, castor oil, contents of the lecithin capsules, and contents of the vitamin E capsule.

2. Prepare the gelatin by dissolving it in the cold water.

3. Add the boiling water to the gelatin mixture. Stir till dissolved and then cool to room temperature.

4. Add ½ cup (125 ml) of the gelatin mixture to the blender. Blend thoroughly and add only enough water to achieve the consistency of a lotion.

5. Pour into a bottle and store in the refrigerator.

To use:

Use for dry or chapped hands.

QUICK AND EASY HAND SMOOTHING LOTION

1 tablespoon (15 ml) glycerin

1 tablespoon (15 ml) rose water

1 tablespoon (15 ml) non-distilled witch hazel extract

3 tablespoons (45 ml) honey

To make:

1. Blend and shake well.

2. Store in the refrigerator.

To use: Pour a small amount into the palm of your hands and gently massage into your hands and fingers.

PERFECT MOISTURIZING HAND CREAM

The proportions of this cream are about 1 part oil base to 1 part water, essential oils, and vitamins. In the oil base ingredients, the proportions should be approximately 2 parts liquid oil to 1 part solid oil. Tap water is not recommended in the water ingredient because it can sometimes introduce bacteria to your cream that results in the growth of mold. If using aloe vera, the cream will be more dense but very moisturizing.

Oil Base Ingredients

3/4 cup (180 ml) apricot oil and/or sweet almond oil

1/2 cup (125 ml) coconut oil and/or cocoa butter

1 teaspoon (5 ml) anhydrous lanolin

1/2 ounce (15 g) grated beeswax

Water, Essential Oils, and Vitamins

2/3 cup (150 ml) distilled water, rose water, or orange flower water

1/3 cup (75 ml) aloe vera gel

A few drops of the essential oil of your choice

Vitamins A and E (optional)

(Thanks to Rosemary Gladstar and Sage Mountain Herbs for sharing this recipe.)

To make:

1. Heat the oil base ingredients over low heat in a double boiler until the solid oils are melted. Stir gently to mix well.

2. Pour the oil mixture into a glass measuring cup and cool to room temperature. The mixture should become thick, creamy, semisolid, and cream-colored. When completely cooled, you are ready for the next step.

3. Place the water, aloe, essential oil, and vitamins in a blender. Turn blender on the highest speed. In a slow, thin drizzle, pour the oil base mixture into the center hole of the blender.

4. When most of the oil base mixture has been added and the cream resembles a butter-cream frosting (you may not need to use all of the oil base mixture), turn off the blender. Do not overbeat. The cream should be rich and thick and continue to thicken as it sets up.

5. Pour into cream jars, label, and store in a cool place.

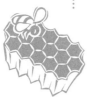

AUBREY'S OLDE ENGLISH LYME-GINSENG MEN'S HAND CREAM

ere is a pungent, heavy-duty hand cream for hard-working hands. It was created just for *Natural Hand Care* by Aubrey Hampton, an herbalist and cosmetic chemist. (You may have seen or tried some of his hair-, skin-, and body-care products under the trade name of Aubrey Organics.) The cream serves as a protective coating and with regular use will improve dry, chapped, and red hands. Although there are 14 ingredients, the recipe is easy to prepare.

1 package (10.5 ounces, or 325 ml) "Silken" tofu (a low-fat soy protein)
1/2 cup (125 ml) organic aloe vera gel
1 tablespoon (15 ml) citrus seed extract
2 tablespoons (30 ml) evening primrose oil
3 tablespoons (45 ml) glycerin
3 tablespoons (45 ml) shea butter
2 tablespoons (30 ml) 100-proof grain alcohol or vodka
12 drops Siberian ginseng tonic (available from Gaia Herbs)
2 drops essential oil of ginger
8 drops essential oil of lemongrass
8 drops essential oil of lemon
2 tablespoons (30 ml) essential oil of lime
6 drops essential oil of grapefruit
1 tablespoon (15 ml) almond oil

To make:

1. Place the tofu into a food blender. Add the aloe vera, citrus seed extract, evening primrose oil, and glycerin. Blend until smooth.

2. Melt the shea butter and add it to the blender ingredients.

3. Add the alcohol; Siberian ginseng tonic; essential oils of ginger, lemongrass, lemon, lime, and grapefruit; and the almond oil. Blend until the mixture becomes smooth.

4. Pour into clean lotion bottles, label, date, and refrigerate.

To use:

Use as needed. When you first apply it, the lemon-lime fragrance will be strong and there will be a bit of a sticky, clingy feeling. In a few moments, the aroma dissipates and the sticky feeling is gone.

UNDERSTANDING INGREDIENTS IN COMMERCIAL SKIN COSMETICS

Chances are that you will not always have the time or energy to make your own hand creams, oils, and salves. For health's sake, it's important to be an informed consumer, and yes, there's one more set of labels to read. These are some of the ingredients to know.

Allantoin

Allantoin is a substance that is soothing and nonirritating to the skin. It stimulates healthy tissue formation and healing of wounds, as well as removes the scales and crusts of dead skin cells. Allantoin has a softening effect on keratin, the protein that is so abundant in the surface cells of the skin, by allowing water to be replenished in the keratin layer. This ingredient is naturally found in the herbs aloe vera, comfrey, and bearberry.

Beneficial Herbs

There are numerous beneficial herbs for hand creams and ointment recipes including aloe, calendula, chickweed, comfrey, viola or garden pansy, plantain, red clover, St.-John's-wort, and yarrow. Many are used as ingredients in commercial hand-care products.

Dead Sea Salt Extract

Dead Sea salt extract, sometimes labeled plain sea salt, naturally increases the skin's ability to retain moisture. Sea salt is an ingredient in some cream moisturizers.

Glycerin

Glycerin is a substance that attracts water but is not easily absorbed, so it will remain on the upper layers of the skin. If 100 percent glycerin is applied as a humectant, it may draw additional moisture from already dry skin. However, since the concentration of glycerin in creams and lotions is usually never more than 50 percent, glycerin can be considered a beneficial ingredient because it improves a cream's spreadability. Glycerin and rose water make a classic formulation that has been used safely for years.

Jojoba

Jojoba extract, commonly known as simply jojoba, is similar to human sebum, the skin's natural restorative fluid. It helps to restore the skin and softens and conditions all skin types. Jojoba is cold-pressed and filtered from the seeds of a desert shrub that is cultivated in dry regions of the world, such as Israel and the Sonoran desert regions of the United States and Mexico.

Jojoba extract is an unusual wax ester with antioxidant and light emollient properties. It rarely turns rancid and does not break down under high temperatures or pressure. Jojoba became an important ingredient for the natural cosmetics industry when it was discovered to imitate the properties of spermaceti oil — a white, crystalline, solid wax from the head of the sperm whale. Spermaceti oil was once used extensively in cosmetics, but has since been banned as a measure of protection for whales. Cetyl alcohol, a form of synthetic spermaceti oil, is an alternative to jojoba, but it can sometimes cause allergic skin reactions.

Lactic Acid

Lactic acid is a natural element of human skin. It is one of the alpha-hydroxy acids that have excellent humectant properties, attracting and retaining moisture. It also helps to maintain the acid balance of the skin.

Lanolin

Lanolin is a fatlike substance produced by oil glands in sheep and obtained from sheep's wool. It can soften dry, chapped, or cracked skin but is also known to cause some allergic sensitivities (approximately 5 percent of the population is allergic to lanolin).

Barrier Oils

Animal, vegetable, and mineral oils help to seal in moisture by forming a slick barrier on the surface of the skin. Mineral oil can be allergenic and clog the skin's pores. Petroleum jelly (petrolatum) is thick and greasy, leaves a heavy film on the skin, and can stain clothing, but does form an effective water and environmental barrier.

Natural oils that are safe and frequently used for skin treatments include oils of sweet almond, apricot kernel, avocado, olive, quince, sesame, sunflower seed, and wheat germ.

Urea

Urea is most often used as a moisturizer in a non-oily base, although it can also function as a preservative. A white, crystalline, water-soluble compound, it is a water-loving (hydrophilic) ingredient. Urea is the end product of both animal and human protein metabolism. If you are allergic to ammonia, you may be allergic to urea in cosmetics.

Preservatives

It would be much simpler if no preservatives were needed in cosmetics, but unless we plan to store all skin products forever in the refrigerator, we have to accept this necessity.

There are two classes of preservatives in beauty aids: antimicrobial agents and antioxidants. Antimicrobial agents, such as alcohol and essential oils, retard the growth of microbacteria and fungi in cosmetics. Antioxidants, such as vitamins A, C, and E and carotene, block oxidation, are free-radical scavengers, and inhibit the destruction of fats and oils.

The FDA requires that the concentration of preservatives in a cosmetic product be sufficiently high to inhibit the growth of microorganisms during its use by the consumer. Without preservatives, a cream or lotion would last only about 8 to 14 days (if refrigerated, about 4 weeks). With commercial preservatives, products can last 2 to 3 years.

Alcohol, essential oils, and vitamins A and E are a few natural preservatives. However, they can be expensive, be volatile, evaporate when uncovered, and sometimes cause skin reddening and dermatitis. Natural cosmetic companies tend to use the least offensive chemical preservatives available to them, such as urea or methyl parabens.

In general, many preservatives are cellular toxins, and I recommend making and using your own fresh, natural cosmetics when possible.

NEW DIRECTIONS IN SKIN COSMETICS

From the old to the new, current technology is bringing the words *phospholipids* and *liposomes* into cosmetic products vocabulary. Phospholipids are part of the fats (lipids) that surround the cells in the stratum corneum, the skin's outermost epidermal layer (see page 19). Their unique structure, consisting of one part that attracts water and two parts that attract lipid substances, forms the outer membrane of all living cells as we know them. These phospholipids play a significant role in helping the skin maintain adequate moisture. Because of environmental influences, we lose phospholipids every day and thus valuable moisture escapes from the skin.

I.R.D. Research Laboratories in Virginia is creating phospholipids outside the body from soy lecithin, a non-animal source. When crammed into a small space, these phospholipids spontaneously form cell-like structures on their own, called liposomes. Instead of being crowded with living cell material, they now contain an empty space that can be occupied with any substance in solution. This capability is revolutionary in its possible impact on delivery systems for cosmetics and medicines.

Using proprietary processes, it is now possible to fill these liposomes with skin cell nutrients such as vitamins and antioxidants. When liposome creams are applied topically, they penetrate deeply to hold moisture and renourish the skin. This is a unique system for skin-care health, and time will be the judge of its efficacy.

CHAPTER 8
Common Skin Ailments:
R_x for the Hands

Tom Sawyer to Huckleberry Finn on how to cure warts:
Dip your hand in a rotten stump filled with rain water and say:
Barley-corn, barley-corn, injun-meal shorts,
Spunk-water, spunk-water, swaller these warts.
— Mark Twain

The skin on your fingers, hands, and arms is subject to many maladies, from allergies to warts. Yet there are easy, natural ways to facilitate healing of bothered skin. Here are possible solutions to these common, troublesome ailments. They are arranged alphabetically by ailment. If you can, opt for the simple remedies first. The body has an amazing capacity to heal itself when we pay attention to its early messages. Should you find that there is little or no improvement within a reasonable amount of time after trying these approaches, seek suitable medical attention.

TESTING FOR SKIN SENSITIVITIES

Any type of skin can become sensitive at some time or another. Whether it is young or mature, oily or dry, skin can be bothered by cosmetics, clothing, chemicals, air pollution, diet, or health changes. Reactions appear as allergic swelling, blemishes, hives, local irritation, or rashes.

Patch-test new cosmetics to find out if your skin is sensitive to certain emulsifiers, detergents, or essential oils. Positive results usually appear as a red, itchy spot. Here's how to test:

Step 1: Use a simple adhesive bandage with a nonstick pad.
Step 2: Saturate the pad of the bandage with the substance to be tested (herb, essential oil, cream, lotion) and place it on your inner forearm.
Step 3: Leave the bandage on for 48 hours unless it causes itching.

Step 4: Remove the bandage and examine your skin with a magnifier.

Step 5: If for any reason your skin begins to itch or hurt, take the patch off immediately, examine the skin, and wash the skin area.

Note: A patch test is not a 100% accurate guarantee that there won't be a reaction somewhere else on your skin.

Allergies

What they are: Allergies are sensitivities to particular substances known as allergens. These substances can be harmless to one person yet deadly to another. Allergic reactions are also not always predictable. A person can experience no reaction in one instance and the next day be exposed to the same substance and break out in hives. (See page 146 for more on hives.)

A healthy body can usually resist allergens. A body under stress or lacking vital nutrients, however, may show a suppressed immune response and leave the door open for foreign substances.

Allergens penetrate the body in various ways. They may be injected as in drugs or vaccines; enter the skin through contact with cosmetics, plants, or other materials; be conveyed by insect bites; be inhaled as pollen or dust; or be absorbed through the foods we eat.

Suggested remedies: The best way to handle contact allergies is to avoid the offending substance. And the part of your body most often used for contact? You guessed it — your hands. So protect yourself by keeping aware of what you touch. Remember, you can have contact with an allergen with one part of your body and have an allergic reaction that shows up in another area of your body. (For instance, at a recent flower show, a vendor was selling a barrier cream against poison ivy. I tried it on my hands and within minutes, my eyes were burning.) Wearing gloves is a reliable defense.

ALLERGIC ALERT

If you experience swelling in your face or lips, have difficulty breathing, or have stomach cramps, you may be experiencing a severe allegic reaction. Call for help immediately.

A second strategy against allergic response is to augment the diet with herbs that stimulate the natural immune system, are anti-inflammatory, and have actions that work to rid the body of alien matter. These plants activate the metabolism and provoke the function of the liver, kidneys, and intestines, the body's major organs of elimination. Some anti-allergy herbs to try are:

- Burdock leaves and root
- Dandelion leaves and root
- Stinging nettles (aerial parts)
- Red clover flower heads
- Parsley leaves (avoid large doses during pregnancy)
- Plantain leaves

These are simply basic approaches to dealing with common allergies. The remedies suggested here are by no means a comprehensive strategy for natural care of this problem. Allergies are a challenging issue well beyond the scope of hand care, and for more information you should consult an allergy specialist.

PERSONAL BLEND HERBAL TEA

To relieve the symptoms of allergies, try using any of the herbs listed above. This tea is an easy method of incorporating them into your diet.

2–3 teaspoons (10–15 ml) fresh herbs or 1 teaspoon (5 ml) crushed dried herbs
1 cup (250 ml) boiling water
Fresh lemon or honey (optional)

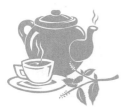

To make:
1. Pour the boiling water over the crushed herbs. You can use more than one herb at a time. Be creative!
2. Cover and steep for 5–10 minutes before drinking.
3. Add fresh lemon or honey to taste.
Note: If you are using bark, roots, or seeds, crush these first to make their contents more accessible and to bring out the flavors. Then boil them in water for 10–15 minutes.
To use:
Drink!

ALLERGY BEGONE TEA

The idea of adding Swedish bitters, a combination of 11 herbs in an alcohol base, to tea is shared by Barbara and Peter Theiss in *The Family Herbal*. Swedish bitters stimulate digestion and help the body remove excess waste products. Elder flowers are immune-system builders, and the raspberry leaves and honey will lessen the bitter taste. Swedish bitters are available at most natural food stores.

1 cup (250 ml) water
3 parts nettles, red clover, or dandelion (choose one or any combination of the three)
1 part raspberry leaves
1 part elder flowers (optional)
Up to 1 teaspoon (5 ml) Swedish bitters (optional)
Honey to taste

To make:

1. Bring the water to a boil, then remove from heat. Blend the nettles, clover, or dandelion together with the raspberry leaves and elder flowers. Steep in the hot water for 5 to 10 minutes.

2. Add the Swedish bitters directly into the teacup or teapot with the honey.

To use:

Drink 1 cup, two or three times a day, until allergy symptoms disappear. Drink 1 cup a day afterward for system maintenance. Don't become so enthusiastic that you overdose on this tea. Two cups a day is adequate, as this tea can act as a diuretic. *Caution:* Avoid high doses of raspberry leaves during early pregnancy; also, see page 233 for cautions about Swedish bitters.

A PERFECT CUP OF HERBAL TEA

A really wonderful product for brewing a single cup of herbal tea is a Swiss-made permanent tea filter called Swiss Gold TF 250. The gold filter fits into an individual teacup, has plenty of room for fresh or dried loose herbs, and has a cover to encourage great brewing. Simply place the filter in the cup, toss in your own combination of herbs, pour in boiling water, cover, and steep for 5 to 10 minutes. You should be able to find Swiss Gold in cookery shops or in stores that specialize in coffee and tea products.

Bee Stings and Bug Bites

Birds sing but bees sting, and so do wasps, yellow jackets, hornets, and fire ants (by injecting poison into our skin), while female mosquitoes and some other insects bite. The only difference in treating the redness, pain, inflammation, and itch of stings versus insect bites is the necessity of scraping out the bee stinger first, so that no more venom is injected. This must be done before any attempt to soothe the skin. Don't remove the stinger with your fingers — this will only release more venom. Instead, gently scrape it away with a credit card or butter knife. Apply an ice cube to the sting to reduce inflammation and pain.

Caution: If after a bite or a sting you experience swelling in your face or lips, have difficulty breathing, or have stomach cramps, you may be experiencing a severe allergic reaction. Call for medical help immediately.

Suggested remedies: The best method of treating stings or bites is to prevent them from happening at all. To lower your chances of being bee-stung, be aware that bees are drawn to bright colors and sweet smells. So save your perfume, candy-coated desserts, and brightly colored nail polish for other than picnic days. On the other hand, mosquitoes prefer warm, dark colors and clothing. They are also attracted to perspiration, sweet perfumes, and women taking birth-control pills or other hormones. Given these somewhat contradictory conditions, it's tough to come up with an acceptable recommendation for avoiding all these flying critters — you'll have to decide which pest is the larger concern.

Quick bite and sting remedies. Here are simple remedies for other types of insect bites and stings:

- For horsefly bites, apply St.-John's-wort oil.
- For ant stings, apply bicarbonate of soda.
- For spider bites, dab on apple cider vinegar or diluted ammonia.
- For wasp stings, pat with apple cider vinegar.

Vitamin C paste. To treat spider bites and insect stings, make a paste of powdered vitamin C mixed with water, and apply directly to the skin.

PENNYROYAL PEST PREVENTION

"Two bugs in the bush are better than one on the hand."

If you or someone you care for is especially sweet (I mean very appealing to mosquitoes or other insects), a potted plant of pennyroyal (*Mentha pulegium* or *Hedeoma pulegioides*), an aromatic member of the Mint family, might just make sitting on the patio or lawn enjoyable again. Both of these varieties are strong, herbal insect repellents and have been used for this purpose for centuries. Just move the plant to wherever you are sitting, and it should discourage buzzing and biting visitors.

BEE STING/BUG BITE TREATMENT

(For bug bites, proceed directly to Step 4.)

Step 1: Scrape away the bee stinger (try using a butter knife or a credit card).

Step 2: If you have a known allergy to bee stings, use an antihistamine immediately or seek prompt medical help.

Step 3: Apply ice to reduce swelling.

Step 4: If you are not allergic to stings but want to relieve the pain, apply the clean leaves of any of the following herbs. These applications can also ease the itch of bug bites.

- ◆ **Basil** (crushed fresh leaves): Rub fresh, crushed leaves on the affected spot to relieve itching and inflammation.
- ◆ **Dandelion:** Apply the white, milky latex from the split stems directly on the sting or bite to soothe the skin.
- ◆ **Onion:** For rapid relief, place fresh slices of onion on insect stings or food-allergy-related hives.
- ◆ **Parsley:** Apply the juice of the plant directly, or use in a compress to reduce swelling.
- ◆ **Plantain:** Rinse or wipe the leaf clean, chew it briefly, then place it on the sting; in less than a minute, you will feel a cooling sensation and notice a lessening of the swelling.
- ◆ **Yellow dock:** Apply fresh macerated leaves to the sting.

WEED WALK

In the summer on Cape Cod, a neighbor and I frequently take a brisk morning walk, slowed only by my persistence in pointing out the wild things that grow that can be used for simple remedies. For some strange reason, on our street, plantain grows only on his property. I extolled the virtues of this weedlike plant in alleviating the pain of bee stings. My busy executive friend placated me by listening, but I did not feel that I had his complete attention.

A month into the summer, his visiting daughter was stung by a bee. A frantic phone call to come and show him again "that weed you said would help" changed his outlook forever. Meeting them on their property, I pointed out *Plantago major*, which his daughter agreed to partially chew and then place on the sting. (She had already removed the bee's stinger.) Almost immediately, she felt a cooling sensation and relief from the uncomfortable bite. Ahh! Vindication is sweet.

STING-EASE OINTMENT

To relieve bee stings or bug bites, you can also make an ointment with yellow dock or plantain. Keep it with you in a first-aid kit when you venture into the field.

1 tablespoon (15 ml) pure beeswax, unbleached

1/3 cup (75 ml) infused oil of yellow dock or plantain leaves (see box On page 124)

Contents of one 400 IU vitamin E capsule

10 drops essential oil of lavender or geranium (optional)

To make:

1. Gently melt the beeswax in a double boiler and carefully add the infused herb oil. Stir to combine.

2. Remove from the heat and cool the mixture.

3. Stir in the contents of the vitamin E capsule and the essential oil of your choice.

4. Pour into small sterile jars (I use 2 one-ounce [30 g] jars).

5. When the mixture is completely cool, seal and label with the ingredients used and the date produced. Store in a cool place.

INFUSING DOCK OR PLANTAIN

To make infused oil, windowsill method: Dry the fresh yellow dock or plantain leaves for a day or two in a shady location. Coarsely chop several handfuls of the dried leaves. Place these in a jar and cover with olive oil. Allow to steep in the oil for 7 to 10 days on a sunny windowsill, turning the jar daily. Strain, bottle, and store in a dark, cool location.

To make infused oil, stove-top method: Put the chopped, fresh herbs in a double boiler and cover with olive oil. Set on the lowest temperature possible and simmer just until the herbs are wilted. (Don't walk away from this process or you'll have fried herbs.) Remove from heat and let cool uncovered. Let this warm mixture rest, covered, for 12 hours. Then strain carefully to remove all plant leaves. Use cheesecloth and strain twice if necessary. The moisture will have separated from the oil. Carefully pour the oil into a double boiler and heat gently. You may notice sprays of droplets "bursting." When these stop occurring, the oil is reasonably free of water content. Let the herb oil cool completely. Pour into a clean bottle, being careful not to disturb any sediment that may be at the bottom of the pot. Cap or cork and label. Store in a dark, cool location.

Blisters

What they are: Friction blisters are localized collections of fluid in the epidermis that cause elevations of the outermost skin layer and separation from the underlying tissue. Blisters are usually caused by friction and sometimes by a burn.

Suggested remedies: You aren't going to believe this, but following are two unlikely remedies for soothing blisters — dandelions and peach pits.

DANDY STEMS FOR BLISTERS

Of all green vegetables, dandelion is one of the best sources of vitamin A (14,000 IU per every 100 g raw). Remember, vitamin A is important in the repair of body tissues. Try this simple approach to soothe a blister:

Thick, succulent dandelion stems

To make:

1. Pick fresh, substantial-size dandelion stems. Be sure they have not been sprayed with pesticides. (Use a field guide for help with identification.)

2. Gently split the stem to get at the sap.

To use:

1. Apply the white, milky juice to the blister.

2. Cover loosely with an adhesive bandage.

Caution: Some people have skin sensitivity to the milky juice in the stems and leaves of the dandelion. If you feel any discomfort, wash off the juice.

PEACH PIT TEA COMPRESS

Peach pits are another remedy for blisters. Enjoy fresh peaches while they are in season, but save the rinsed and dried pits in a labeled jar.

2 peach pits
1 cup (250 ml) boiling water

To make:

1. Simmer the peach pits for 10 minutes in the boiling water. The water will take on a reddish hue.

2. Cool the liquid until comfortable to the skin and pour ½ cup of the peach tea water onto a clean cotton cloth.

To use:

Apply as a compress to the blister for 10–15 minutes. Repeat as needed. Leftover liquid should be refrigerated between uses.

Boils

What they are: Boils, also known as furuncles, are uncomfortable, hard swellings arising from infections of hair follicles and sweat glands that usually appear on the wrist, forearm, or the cap of the elbow. A boil can form when the skin tissue is weakened by chafing or injury, or when there is lowered body resistance to infection because of disease or inadequate nutrition. The nodule has a central core of pus surrounded by inflamed and swollen tissue. Itching and mild pain can also accompany a boil.

Suggested remedies: There are a couple of ways to treat boils naturally. Keeping the area around the boil scrupulously clean is number one. If the boil does not improve in two or three days, consult a healthcare practitioner.

- Boils can spread, so if you have one, take showers instead of baths so that the bacterial infection does not spread to other parts of the body.
- Wear disposable gloves and wash hands frequently when touching and disposing of the soiled gauze dressings.
- Eat foods rich in vitamins A, C, and E and zinc, or add these supplements to your diet (see chapter 3 for more information).
- Drink hot water with lemon juice or make nettle, red clover, or burdock tea to cleanse the system.
- Begin to dose with a dropperful of echinacea extract, an immune-system enhancer, in water three times a day.
- Use warm compresses and topical antiseptic treatment to disinfect and speed healing.

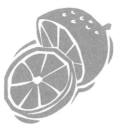

LINSEED OR FLAX COMPRESS FOR BOILS

Dr. Rudolph Fritz Weiss recommends linseed compresses, made from the seed of the flax plant, to bring a boil on the skin to a head.

2 small linen or muslin
    bags
Linseed (also known as
    flax seed; available in
    health food stores)
Essential oil of lavender or
    tea tree

To make:

1. Fill two small linen bags one-third full of linseeds, and then sew the ends of the bags closed.

2. Fill a large pot with water and bring it to a rolling boil.

3. Drop the first bag in the boiling water and simmer for 10 minutes. The seeds will swell to fill the bag.

4. Remove the hot linen bag with a ladle and place it in a large strainer over the sink. Carefully press out the excess water.

To use:

1. Wrap the bag in a clean cloth and place the compress on the boil as hot as can be tolerated. Put the second bag in the boiling water so that one bag can be exchanged for another as they cool.

2. Apply the linseed compresses at least twice a day until the infection comes to a head.

3. Once the boil has opened, a few drops of essential oil of lavender or tea tree oil, with antibacterial and anti-inflammatory properties, can be applied to the sterile dressing before covering the wound. Change this dressing three times a day to keep the wound clean and dry.

Bruises

What they are: Bruises, or "black-and-blue" marks, usually come from an impact that causes bleeding in small blood vessels beneath the skin. Those with fragile skin or bleeding disorders and people taking aspirin, estrogen, or cortisone-type medications may be more susceptible to bruising.

There are a variety of natural and herbal remedies for treating bruises — some for external application (see below) and others for internal ingestion (see page 131). Read through the selections before deciding on the remedy that's best for you.

Suggested external remedies: Compresses and creams are common and effective external preparations for treating bruises.

Arnica tincture compress. Arnica affects the circulation. It is used to reduce inflammation and the signs of bruising by increasing the body's ability to prevent the escape of blood into bruised tissue. It breaks the blood clot into smaller segments.

You can use a diluted alcohol tincture of crushed arnica flowers in a compress, diluting 1 tablespoon (15 ml) of the tincture in 8 ounces (240 ml) of cool water. Wet a cloth and apply to "black-and-blue" fingers, hands, or arms. Do *not* use on broken skin — arnica prevents the blood from clotting, and it may cause the open wound to bleed. Witch hazel is also a good complement to arnica (see page 203).

Caution: Those taking blood thinners or who have blood disorders should check with their physician before using arnica.

Aloe gel. The value of aloe vera lies in its ability to regenerate damaged tissues. Although it is often prescribed for use on healing wounds to prevent scarring, aloe also functions as an analgesic for mild pain. If you have a windowsill, it's worth keeping an aloe plant in your home. To use the fresh plant, cut off a lower leaf near the central stalk, split the leaf lengthwise, remove the gel, and apply directly to the affected area.

Calendula ointment. Calendula has provitamin A, or carotenoids (similar to what is in carrots), that act to restore the skin's own powers of recovery. Use calendula ointment (which can be found in most herb shops or natural food stores) or oil (see recipe on page 129) anywhere on the skin. You can also use calendula on open wounds.

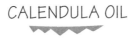

CALENDULA OIL

Calendula officinalis, also known as pot marigold, is a sun-loving Mediterranean plant with yellow and deep orange flowerheads. It contains both beta carotene and vitamin C, and is used in many skin-soothing preparations, including oils, tinctures, creams, ointments, and even talc. It is particularly useful for chapped or cracked hands.

1 cup (250 ml) dried calendula flowers

2 cups (500 ml) cold-pressed oil (olive, sweet almond, apricot, sesame, sunflower, or walnut)

Note: You can also make this oil with fresh calendula flowers. In this case, fill the jar with loosely packed flowers and steep in oil for only about 3 to 4 weeks. Once filtered, let the oil sit for 24 hours and then remove any sludge or particulates that may have settled to the bottom of the container with a poultry baster.

To make:

1. Fill a clean glass jar to within an inch of the top with the dried flowers. Then gently pack the flowers down with a spoon.

2. Slowly pour most of the oil into the jar, making sure that it completely covers the flowers. Stir gently with a non-metal utensil (I use a wooden chopstick) to remove any air bubbles. Then top off with the remaining oil and seal the jar with a lid or a double layer of cheesecloth secured with a rubber band.

3. Place the jar in a paper bag and set on a warm, sunny windowsill for 5 to 6 weeks. Turn the jar weekly and inspect for moisture. If there is moisture, open the jar, carefully wipe it off with a clean towel, and reseal.

4. When the oil is a beautiful golden color, it is ready. Strain through a cheesecloth to remove the flowers. Then strain again through a paper coffee filter to remove any smaller debris.

5. Pour the oil into clean jars, seal, and label. Store in a cool dark place and use within one year.

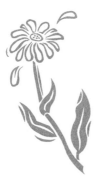

MARIGOLD PETAL AND
COMFREY CREAM FOR BRUISING

Both the leaf and the root of comfrey are used to promote rapid healing. The leaves have a high content of mucilage and allantoin, which stimulate cell division in the epidermis. The root is rich in vitamin B_{12}.

2 tablespoons (30 ml) fresh, mature comfrey leaf, or 1 tablespoon dried

1 cup (250 ml) boiling water

1 tablespoon (15 ml) beeswax

1 tablespoon (15 ml) lanolin or shea butter

1 tablespoon (15 ml) cocoa butter or jojoba

1½ tablespoons (23 ml) calendula oil (see recipe on page 129)

1 teaspoon (5 ml) glycerin

¼ teaspoon (1 ml) borax

6 drops essential oil of sweet orange zest (or your choice)

Yield: Makes two 1-ounce (30 g) jars

(Adapted from a recipe by Lesley Bremness.)

To make:

1. Crush the comfrey leaves with a rolling pin and cover with the boiling water. Simmer gently for 10 minutes. Strain the leaves from the infused liquid.

2. Melt the beeswax, then add the lanolin or shea butter and cocoa butter or jojoba. Stir occasionally to hasten melting and blend with the beeswax.

3. Add the calendula oil and glycerin and slowly stir into the beeswax mixture. Remove from heat.

4. Dissolve the borax in the warm comfrey infusion and stir 2 tablespoons (30 ml) into the beeswax mixture.

5. Continue stirring this mixture until it becomes thick and begins to cool. Mix in the essential oil.

6. Spoon into jars. Fill around the edges first and then fill in the middle. Cap and label with the ingredients and date. Keep refrigerated.

To use:

Clean the surface of the bruise. Using a small spatula to remove the cream from the jar, gently apply to the bruised area. Repeat every morning and evening until the bruise has healed.

Suggested internal remedies: While it may seem surprising, there are several supplements you can take internally to help your body recover quickly from a bruise. These supplements increase circulation and break down or prevent the pooling of blood underneath the skin that creates the visible bruise.

Vitamin C supplements. At the first sign of a bruise, it's vitamin C to the rescue. Take 500 to 1000 mg daily to reduce bleeding under the skin.

Ginkgo biloba extract. A standardized extract of the leaves of this tree, one of the oldest species in the world, will improve circulation to the hands and feet and also speed healing. One of its constituents, gingkolide B, inhibits blood platelet clumping and will work to break down the bruise. You can find ginkgo biloba extract in most herb shops or natural food stores.

Hawthorn extract. An extract of the berries and flowers of hawthorn dilates coronary arteries, lowers blood pressure, increases circulation, and helps break down bruises. You can find hawthorn extract in most herb shops or natural food stores. The basic dose is 30 drops of the extract, two to three times a day, as long as needed. You may also make a tea using 1 to 2 teaspoons (5–10 ml) of the dried herb infused in 1 cup (250 ml) boiling water.

Minor Burns, Scalds, and Sunburn

What they are: Burns are graded by the severity of their impact on the skin. First-degree burns show redness, but do not break the skin. Second-degree burns show redness and blistering. Third- and fourth-degree burns cause a change in texture of the skin because of the death of cells at various layers of the skin. We will be dealing only with first- and, potentially, second-degree burns in this section. More severe burns are beyond the scope of this book and require immediate medical attention.

Suggested remedies: There are three things you want to accomplish in treating a burn: reduce pain, prevent infection, and encourage the regeneration of tissue. The very first thing to do with any burn is to cool the affected area to prevent the wound from reaching deeper into the tissue. Rub an ice cube or run cold water over the burn for several minutes. Then you can try applying any of the following preparations.

Yogurt. Apply plain yogurt to inflamed skin as a soothing and cooling remedy. Choose an organic yogurt that is without gelatin and specifies the bacterial cultures in the product — *Lactobacillus acidophilus* or *Lactobacillus Bulgaricus,* for example. Allow the yogurt to remain on the burned region for 5 to 10 minutes or as long as it feels comfortable. Then rinse with water that has been boiled and cooled, and pat dry with a clean cloth.

Aloe gel. Spread a thin layer of aloe vera gel from a fresh aloe leaf or a commercial pure gel on the affected area. If necessary, dilute the gel with distilled water.

Honey. If you don't have aloe gel available, honey can be used as a substitute.

Apple cider vinegar dilution. Pat a cool apple cider vinegar mixture on sunburned hands and arms. Prepare a clean bottle with 1 part vinegar to 6 parts distilled water. Repeat the application every 20 minutes.

Green tea compress. Make a big pot of green tea and dilute with cool, distilled water. Lay clean, tea-soaked, cotton cloth compresses on the sunburned skin.

Chamomile and lavender infusion. Both lavender flowers and German chamomile are antimicrobial and mildly sedative. Make an infusion (tea) of German chamomile and lavender flowers using a large pinch of chamomile and a large pinch of lavender to a quart (liter) of water. Adjust the amount of each herb to taste. Drink up to four cups of tea a day.

Macerated gingerroot. Mash fresh gingerroot to release its juices, then apply to the burned area. Those who have tried this remedy report that relief is instantaneous and that a single application is enough to ease the pain of minor burns.

COOL POTATO BURN RELIEF

A burn pulls moisture from the skin. Applying fresh slices of potato to the burn is very cooling, and the skin will "drink" in the moisture. In addition, when I have used this remedy, I've had very little scarring after the burn had healed.

1 raw potato

To make:
Peel a raw potato and cut it into thin slices, or pulp it with a hand grater or food processor.
To use:
1. Apply the potato slices or raw pulp to soothe minor burns, an itchy rash, or bruises.
2. Apply fresh slices or pulp as each becomes dry.

LAVENDER FLOWER WASH

This infusion of lavender will help soothe and reduce redness and inflammation. Lavender also helps inhibit bacteria.

¼ cup (60 ml) fresh or dried lavender flowers
2 cups (500 ml) distilled water
½ tablespoon (8 ml) tincture of benzoin (available at most pharmacies) or 10 drops essential oil of lavender (optional)

To make:
1. Bruise the flowers with the back of a flat wooden paddle.
2. Simmer the flowers gently in distilled water (to cover) for 20 minutes or place in a covered jar with distilled water in a sunny window for an afternoon.
3. Strain through cheesecloth and store in a closed glass bottle in the refrigerator.
4. If you do not plan to use the flower water within a few days, add tincture of benzoin or 10 drops of essential oil of lavender. Shake well.
To use:
Pat on burn and repeat as necessary.

Chapped, Cracked, Red, Rough Hands

What it is: There are various opinions about the causes of chapped skin. The most logical explanation is overexposure of the hands to cold weather or low dew points (humidity). Another cause of chapping is repeated washing of the hands with harsh detergents. This not only chaps the hands but also allows fissuring so that contact irritants can gain entrance to the skin. Dry, chapped skin can also be one of the first signs of a vitamin A deficiency.

Suggested remedies: The most obvious remedy for chapped, cracked hands is moisturizer — and lots of it! There are several recipes listed below. However, you also want to find out why your hands are becoming so dry and chapped. If constant washing or overexposure is necessary given your job or living circumstances, moisturizer may be your only hope (although you should certainly wear gloves whenever possible). However, it may be that you suffer from a vitamin deficiency or you haven't been caring for your hands, in which case you should take preventive measures to guard against painfully cracked hands.

Vitamin therapy. One of the first signs of a vitamin A deficiency may be continually dry or chapped hands. Are carrots, sweet potatoes, and tomatoes on the menu? Do you have sandpaper skin or "gooseflesh" on the outer aspect of your arms and legs that does not go away? If you have these bumps on the outside of your thighs, check with your healthcare practitioner about the possibility of taking daily vitamin A supplements.

If you have been on a stringent diet and eliminated most fats from your menu, you may also be lacking in vitamin E. Add 2 tablespoons (30 ml) daily of wheat germ or an unsaturated oil like corn oil — both of which are rich in vitamin E — to your diet. Once your skin returns to its soft, lovable self, you can gradually reduce the amount of oil or wheat germ.

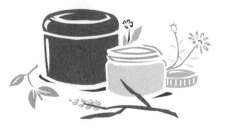

SPECIAL WASH FOR CHAPPED HANDS

This is a gentle cleanser that should not be irritating to the skin. If you repeat this regimen day and night several times a week, your chapped hands will become a thing of the past.

(The cornmeal accomplishes by a gentle abrasive action what a harsh soap does by chemical action. The cornmeal, however, does not draw all the moisture away from the important lower layers of the skin.)

1 small cucumber
1/2 tablespoon (8 ml) honey
Warm water
Mild soap — fine castile or Dove or Neutrogena
1 tablespoon (15 ml) cornmeal

To make:

1. Peel the cucumber and remove the seeds; blend or juice the vegetable for a few seconds. Mix with the honey and set aside in a small bowl.

2. Make a cornmeal paste by mixing warm water, soap, and cornmeal.

To use:

1. Wash your hands thoroughly with the cornmeal paste. Then rinse hands well in clean, warm (not hot) water. This helps to remove flaking skin cells and any soluble environmental pollutants.

2. While your hands are damp, apply the cucumber juice and honey mixture. Have someone help you wrap your hands in plastic wrap or insert them in large, zip-seal plastic bags. Cover with a towel, then relax as long as possible.

3. Rinse and dry hands. Apply moisture cream. If you've done this at night, wear loose-fitting cotton gloves to bed. (Wash the gloves regularly.)

4. Repeat this cornmeal wash daily (and repeat as often as you can for badly chapped hands). In cold weather, substitute a *cold* water rinse in the morning to acclimate the hands to cooler conditions. Dry well and then rub in a moisturizing cream.

ALMONDS, COMFREY, AND
HONEY SOOTHING OINTMENT

Here is a recipe from the Middle Ages for painfully cracked hands.

Almonds are known for their mildness and softening action on the skin. Comfrey, also known as bruisewort or knitbone, has been cultivated in gardens for centuries for the wound-healing qualities of the root and leaves. Allantoin, one of the constituents of comfrey, encourages healthy skin regrowth by stimulating cells, and also relieves itching.

1 ounce (30 g) ground almonds
1 egg, beaten
1/4 ounce (7 g) ground comfrey root
1 tablespoon (15 ml) honey

To make:
Combine well the almonds, egg, comfrey root, and honey, stirring with your hands or a wooden spoon. Refrigerate. (Of course, they didn't have refrigerators in the Middle Ages.)

To use:
1. Before bed, smooth this mixture over your hands and fingers and pull on either a pair of cotton gloves or old leather gloves. Follow this regimen for seven nights.
2. Each morning, rinse your hands and the gloves and apply a skin lotion. After the nightly routine of the first week, cut back to a once-a-week schedule for a month, and then repeat this recipe only on a monthly basis.
Caution: Internal use of comfrey is not recommended.

RED HANDS TIP

You can whiten red hands by rubbing them several times a day with a mixture of egg white and glycerin. At night, wear gloves to bed.

CHATHAM CHAP CREAM

This is a two-step recipe that involves first preparing an infused oil and then using the oil to prepare the cream. It's a wonderfully soothing moisturizer for chapped skin on the hands and around the nails.

Step 1: The Oil

1 ounce (30 g) dried lavender blossoms

1 ounce (30 g) dried comfrey leaf

1 ounce (30 g) dried chamomile flowers

1 ounce (30 g) dried calendula flowers

1 ounce (30 g) dried goldenseal leaf or Oregon grape root

Almond oil or olive oil to cover

Step 2: The Cream

1/2 ounce (15 g) beeswax

2/3 cup (150 ml) infused herb oil (from Step 1)

1/3 cup (75 ml) coconut oil

3/4 cup (180 ml) distilled water

1/4 cup (60 ml) fresh aloe gel (or aloe extract with natural gum)

Contents of two 400 IU vitamin E capsules

Yield: Makes eight 2-ounce (60 g) jars

(Shared by herbalist Sandy Collingwood, co-founder and owner of Chatham Herbary, Chatham, Massachusetts.)

To make oil:

Place all five dried herbs in a large jar, cover with oil, and seal. Place in a sunny window for two to three weeks. Strain twice through cheesecloth and pour into a clean jar. Seal and label until ready to make the cream. Store in a cool place.

To make cream:

1. Gently melt the beeswax in a saucepan. Add the infused herb and coconut oils. Stirring constantly, heat just enough to liquefy, but do not boil.

2. Pour this mixture into a glass measuring cup and cool to room temperature (10 to 20 minutes).

3. In a blender, combine the distilled water and aloe gel. Blend until thick.

4. Add the cooled oil and beeswax mixture to the aloe water. Blend in short pulses. If the beeswax is too warm, it will separate. If this happens, pour the water off and let cool until you can try again.

5. Add the contents of the vitamin E capsules. Blend and pour into 2-ounce (60 g) jars with lids. Label and date the cream. Keep refrigerated.

Note: Goldenseal is now considered an endangered plant. If you purchase this herb, ask your supplier to verify that it was obtained responsibly.

Here are two 17th-century remedies for "chops in the hands" that offer a unique use for common garden ingredients:

Slugs and Snails and Puppy-Dog Tails

"Chafing of the skin is instantly relieved by the slime of a slug. Put the slug on the sore place; it heals you, and you need not hurt it; the part once slimed the slug may be let go."

Lady Honeywood's "Snail-Water"

"Take a quart of shelled snails, wash them in salt, and water, then scalld them in boyling water; then distill them in a quart of milk upon white sugar candy, and a branch of speremint."

— From W.T. Fernie, M.D., *Meals Medicinal with "Herbal Simples,"* 1905.

Eczema

What it is: A form of dermatitis, eczema is one of the most common and troublesome of inflammatory skin ailments. Eczema is thought to be caused by internal metabolic disturbances or external irritants. It can occur at any stage of life and anywhere on the body, including the hands, wrists, the bend of the elbow, or anywhere else on the arm.

Eczema is characterized by redness, flaking, and blistering of the skin. These bumps begin to cluster, forming very small blisters that fill with clear, colorless fluid and then burst, leaving the skin cracked, itchy, crusty or scaly, and weepy, with possible bleeding.

Allergic eczema may run in families together with hay fever, asthma, and chronic sinus infections. Scratching makes this eczema worse. You can see allergic eczema on the hands and at the bend of the elbows.

Discoid or nummular eczema has coin-shaped disks of red, flaking, weeping, and itching skin, and is most commonly seen on the arms and legs. The cause is unknown.

Contact eczema or dermatitis is caused by a reaction to certain substances that touch the skin. The skin becomes red and itchy, even after contact, and tiny blisters may develop. The tiny blisters sometimes join to form large blisters that break, scale, and crust over. Harsh detergents, chemicals, and poisonous plants are potential culprits. Repetitive friction from a hammer, screwdriver, or other tool may activate contact dermatitis. Rinsing the skin and applying a calendula ointment (available at most herb shops or natural food stores) or comfrey preparation (such as the Almond, Comfrey, and Honey Soothing Ointment on page 136) can be soothing and help to relieve redness and irritation.

Suggested Remedies: Here are some handy tips, recommended by Dr. Stephen M. Schleicher, a Philadelphia dermatologist, to speed healing from eczema or dermatitis:

- Wash your hands in only *lukewarm* water with a mild, unscented soap.
- Avoid direct contact with detergents, polishes, solvents, and stain removers (try wearing gloves for cleaning projects). Anything that removes the natural oil from the skin makes the eczema worse.
- Wear cotton-lined, water-repellent gloves when you shampoo or apply hair dye.
- Use gloves when you peel or squeeze citrus fruits.
- Bypass rings on your fingers when doing housework.
- Rely on cotton-lined gloves for household tasks. Keep them clean inside and out. Wash the gloves several times a week.
- Be cautious about chemicals and other possible skin irritants for at least four or five months after the dermatitis has healed. Prevention is the best medicine.

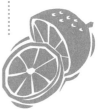

Diet. Physicians disagree, but some think food allergies may play a role in the causes of eczema. Allergic reactions to dairy foods, eggs, wheat products, oranges, and chocolate may trigger outbreaks of this unpleasant skin condition. If you want to experiment, remove each of the foods from your diet for one month. If it makes no difference in the condition of your skin, add it back. Also, add to your menu once or twice a week foods that contain essential fatty acids, such as mackerel, sardines, and salmon. Include garlic, onion, carrots, lettuce, grapes, lemon juice, and dandelion greens in your diet. Everyone is biochemically different and will respond uniquely to each of these options.

Nutritional supplements. Add vitamins A, B complex, and E, plus magnesium and lecithin. Then add the essential fatty acids from evening primrose oil or borage oil along with zinc.

Whey concentrate. Dr. H.C. Alfred Vogel, a noted naturopath, has treated eczema with direct application of undiluted whey concentrate in combination with lactic acid. For stubborn cases, he prepares a compress of Molkosan — a homeopathic whey concentrate — which he soaks in absorbent cotton and binds on the affected lesions. The hand or arm is then encased in a plastic-wrap dressing overnight. Whey concentrate can also be taken internally when diluted with water. Look for whey concentrate in health or nutrition stores that stock homeopathic remedies.

Oatmeal bath. An oatmeal bath can also help to relieve dry, itchy skin. (See recipe for Oatmeal Hand Bath on page 147.)

Vitamin B$_6$ skin salves. A natural skin salve that includes vitamin B$_6$ is also recommended for healing eczema. Use these salves several times during the day, and with cotton gloves at night.

Burdock oil. Apply burdock oil several times a day. (See Burdock Seed Nail and Cuticle Conditioner recipe on page 70.)

BURDOCK WASH

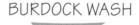

Burdock makes a soothing wash for irritated skin caused by eczema.

2 pinches fresh or dried burdock leaves
1 quart (1 liter) water
Chopped, fresh onion for use with dried burdock leaves (optional)

To make:

1. Blanch the burdock leaves in boiling water. If the leaves are fresh, boil about 10 minutes, or until they are limp.

2. If the leaves of the burdock are dried, moisten them in boiling water. In a separate bowl, mix equal parts of chopped fresh onion with the dried burdock leaves.

To use:

Spread the limp leaves, as hot as you can comfortably handle, on the bothered skin.

1888 ECZEMA LOTION

A recipe from *The Practical Home Physician* by Lyman et al., 1888, offers an easy-to-prepare lotion for eczema lesions.

1 dram (1 teaspoon; 5 ml) borax
2 drams (2 teaspoons; 10 ml) carbonate of soda
2 ounces (1 wineglass; 65 ml) glycerin
4 ounces (1 teacup; 130 ml) distilled water

Mix all ingredients well. Apply lotion to a linen patch, and then lay linen over affected skin.

HORSETAIL COMPRESS

Horsetail is also an effective remedy for treating the symptoms of eczema and psoriasis.

1 teaspoon (5 ml) dried or fresh crushed horse-tail herb stems
1 cup (250 ml) water

To make:
1. Boil ingredients together for 10–15 minutes.
2. To make a compress for bothered skin, place a soft, clean cotton dish towel in the boiled, cooled herb water.
3. Squeeze out excess liquid.
To use:
1. Wrap cloth around hands.
2. Cover with another dry, heavy towel. Allow this compress to remain wrapped around the hands for 10 minutes.

Freckles or Sun Damage

What it is: A freckle is a brownish, pigmented spot on the skin usually caused by exposure to ultraviolet light.

Suggested remedies: To lighten freckles, try any of these options:

- Use buttermilk wash to lighten sun-damaged spots.
- Rub peeled, ripe cucumber slices on freckled hands or arms (this is a passed-down, "grandma" recipe).
- Pat a mixture of lemon juice and honey on freckles. It's great for your skin.
- Sorrel leaves are used in China to fade sun-induced spots. Make a compress of chopped fresh sorrel leaves on a strip of folded gauze. Leave on the skin for fifteen minutes. Repeat every two or three days.

ELDER FLOWER FRECKLE WASH

An elder flower wash is another remedy to lighten freckles and soften the skin.

1 cup (250 ml) fresh
   elder flowers
Distilled water (enough to
   cover the elder flowers)

To make:

1. Cover elder flowers with distilled water and allow to stand overnight.

2. Strain, bottle, and label. Keep refrigerated.

To use:

Bathe the freckles morning and night.

EXTREME FRECKLE REMEDY

This remedy for freckles is not for everyone. It comes from a grandmother in the mountain area of France, from M.F.K. Fisher's *A Cordial Water.*

Take a wineglass of urine and mix it with a tablespoon of good vinegar. Add a pinch of salt. Let it sit for 24 hours. Pat this liquid on freckled skin and leave it on for 30 minutes. Rinse with plain, cold water.

MRS. LEYEL'S LEMON-EGG SKIN TREATMENT

An olde-tyme recipe to keep the hands smooth and fair. This is a gentle skin lightener and bleach that is useful for smoothing and lightening both freckles and brown spots.

White of 1 egg
Freshly squeezed lemon
    juice
2–4 drops essential oil of
    your choice: lavender,
    geranium, or rosemary,
    for example

To make:

1. Measure separately, for equal parts, the white of an egg and the same amount of freshly squeezed lemon juice.

2. In a small earthenware bowl, beat the egg white until stiff. Slowly fold in the lemon juice.

3. Pour into a small pot and warm on the stovetop until the mixture becomes thick, stirring constantly. Scent with the essential oil of your choice.

4. Cool to a comfortable skin temperature.

To use:

1. Dab on hands with cotton squares.

2. Use immediately or store in the refrigerator up to one week. (You may need to rewhip the mixture.)

Frostbite

What it is: Frostbite is a localized cold injury characterized by freezing of the tissues, with ice crystals forming in the cells. Fingers and hands are common sites of frostbite.

The hands and the feet are the farthest from the heart and don't have large, heat-producing muscles. When the body needs to conserve warmth, the peripheral or outer blood vessels are the first to constrict, reducing the blood supply to the hands and feet. This process damages normal circulation so that the skin begins to freeze. Freezing of the tissues extracts water from within the cells and leads to cell dehydration, chemical imbalance, and further obstruction of the blood supply.

The signs of frostbite are usually sensations of cold and pain and a change in color of the hands from very pale to a dull purple (because of poor circulation). Later, as tissues begin to freeze, people lose all sensation.

Suggested remedies: The first step is, as always, prevention. To keep frostbite from happening, be prepared for severe weather conditions. Wear protective clothing and insulated gloves or mittens. (Mittens are preferable because they keep the fingers close together for natural warmth.) Keep your gloves on.

However, regardless of the protections you might take, when there are below-freezing temperatures and significant windchill factors, you are more susceptible to frostbite, especially if:

◆ You are not dressed warmly, not wearing gloves, or using poorly insulated gloves.
◆ Your skin is moist.
◆ Your unprotected skin has contact with frozen metal, such as car-door latches, mailboxes, and metal ice cube trays.
◆ You are a smoker. (Smoking constricts the blood vessels and may make you more sensitive to cold injuries.)
◆ You consume alcohol. (Alcohol numbs the sensation of coldness.)

EMERGENCY FROSTBITE CARE

Step 1: If you're still out in the field, remove any finger rings, watchbands, and constrictive clothing. Do *not* rub the affected area. If there is no sensitivity to aspirin, give one or two aspirin to thin the blood and ease the pain.

Step 2: First warm the central torso of the body. Second, immerse the affected limbs for a *rapid* rewarming of the hands. Prepare a large water bath where you can control the temperature (100 to 108°F; 38 to 42°C) and the person can be warmed and maintained at a normal body temperature. This can be very painful, so try to warm the affected body part in clothing or with another person's body heat first. Ideally, this procedure should be carried out in a hospital. Warming can take 30 to 60 minutes, until the skin tissues are soft and pliable. When the body is cold, the blood vessels in the extremities constrict. If there is no available thermometer, the water temperature should be comfortable (not hot) to a noninjured person's hand.

Step 3: Add warm water as the water cools. Have the person with frostbite remove his or her hands from the bath as warm water is added and stirred into the tub. A sign that the skin is thawing is that hands will take on a flushed appearance. This will be a painful process.

Step 4: Keep injured hands elevated and protected from trauma. Gently place sterile gauze or cotton between the frostbitten fingers to absorb moisture.

Step 5: Do not puncture any blisters that occur — blisters reduce the risk of infection.

Step 6: No smoking! (Smoking constricts the blood vessels, impeding circulation and making it difficult for the damaged tissues to recover.) It can take up to 45 days after cold exposure to assess the extent of damage to the tissues.

Step 7: See a physician as soon as possible.

What they are: Anyone can suffer from hives, which seem to be an allergic reaction to a variety of substances. Very often hives are related to something you ate, such as shellfish, nuts, food additives, or particular medicines. Exact causes are difficult to pinpoint unless hives occur immediately after you have eaten a certain food, taken medicine, or handled a specific thing. In general, there is still a bit of mystery concerning triggers or causes of this skin condition.

Hives are usually red, itchy lumps of variable size on the skin. Sometimes they have a pale center and often they occur in irregular patches. Hives can show up anywhere on the body. They will usually disappear in a few hours but may remain for days or even longer.

Suggested remedies: In most cases, hives are distressing but harmless. There are several simple remedies for easing the itch and soothing the rash, but if the hives persist, or more serious allergic-type reactions occur (see page 118), consult a physician.

AMISH CLEANSING TEA

Generally, if you are experiencing hives you will want to flush out the offending substances. This tea will help, with its mild diuretic effect.

½ teaspoon (2.5 ml) red clover blossoms, dried
1 teaspoon (5 ml) fresh parsley, or ½ teaspoon (2.5 ml) dried
½ teaspoon (2.5 ml) dried nettles
1 cup (250 ml) boiling water

(Adapted from a recipe of Judith Benn Hurley.)

To make:
Put the herbs in a strainer and pour the boiling water over them. Cover and steep the tea for 5 minutes.

To use:
Strain and drink.

Caution: Avoid therapeutic doses of parsley if you are pregnant or nursing. Also, avoid nettles if you have high blood pressure.

MINT TEA CUBES

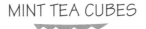

This is a very cooling and soothing remedy and should help to lessen the itch of hives.

2 teaspoons (10 ml) crushed, fresh mint leaves, such as applemint or spearmint, or 1 teaspoon (5 ml) dried
1 cup (250 ml) boiling water

To make:
1. Brew some potent mint tea using 2 teaspoons of fresh mint (or 1 teaspoon dried) per cup of boiling water.
2. Steep for 5 minutes. Strain, if desired.
3. Pour the tea into ice cube trays and freeze. When frozen, transfer the cubes to a plastic freezer bag and label.

To use:
Rub a peppermint cube across your hands or arms to cool itchy hives or irritated skin.

OATMEAL HAND BATH

Oats are not just for horses — for hundreds of years, they've been known to be nutritive, to provide soothing relief for external itching, and to act as a general healing agent for the skin. Today, you can make an oatmeal hand and arm bath to ease hives or eczema.

½ cup (125 ml) oats, ground to a fine powder in a blender (or use oat bran)
Powdered skim milk mixed with boiled water to equal 1 quart (1 liter)
Aloe vera gel (fresh, if possible)

To make:
Combine the warm milk with the oatmeal. Stir until dissolved.

To use:
1. Soak and coat itchy skin with the oatmeal bath.
2. Rinse and pat the skin dry, and apply aloe vera gel over the affected skin.

Itchy Hands

What it is: How does an itch start? This sounds like a simple question, but the answer is not certain. It is believed that the perception of an itch occurs in free nerve endings that lie at the junction of two skin layers — the dermis and the epidermis. Nerve fibers then transmit the sensation to the thalamus, the main relay center in the brain for sensory impulses.

There are at least three main causes of itch: environmental factors, such as bug bites, mites, allergies, strong detergents, and chemicals (baker's itch can result from exposure to yeast and bleaching agents in flour); ailments, such as chicken pox, eczema, and hives; and systemic diseases that affect the whole body, such as Hodgkin's disease and kidney and liver disease.

There seem to be two different types of itch sensations:

♦ A sharp, localized itch that you can satisfy by scratching
♦ A diffuse, spread-out type of itch that is not easily solved by scratching

How does scratching help? It's not well understood. One theory is that scratching overloads the nerve endings so that they cannot simultaneously transmit the itch sensation. Other investigators relate itching to a form of pain. People who can't feel pain don't experience itching. For natural care for itchy hands or arms, see the sections below; for itches related to particular ailments, see the entry for that ailment.

Suggested remedies for environmentally caused itches: These preparations will alleviate itching caused by allergies, scratchy clothes, harsh detergents, chemicals, and insect bites.

Baking soda paste. Rinse the skin. Apply a paste of baking soda and water. Rinse again with cool water. Pat dry.

Chickweed bath or compress. Chickweed will cool, soothe, and relieve irritations and itchiness. Pulverize fresh chickweed to a juice and add to a bath, or use in a compress (see page 157). A Swiss herbalist, Father John Künzle, recommends collecting enough chickweed to boil as you would spinach, and then straining and drinking the juice.

Angelica wash. Make a wash of the leaves of angelica. Pour boiling water over the leaves and let them steep for 15 minutes. Cool the liquid and pat the herbal water on the itchy area.

Witch hazel. For bug-bite itch, dab a solution of non-distilled witch hazel extract alone or with a drop or two of essential oil of tea tree on the irritated area.

Suggested remedies for skin disease itches: These preparations will ease itches caused by systemic diseases such as jaundice and kidney disease.

Cool bath. Lower skin temperature with a cool bath.

Milk or cornstarch wash. Dip a clean cotton cloth in cold skim milk or a mixture of cornstarch and water, and apply to the affected area.

Avoid alcohol. In general, keep away from alcohol because it can increase itching.

Paper Cut

What it is: A paper cut is just what you'd expect — a cut made by paper. It almost always happens to our hands. Although a paper cut is only a minor skin injury, because it allows the escape of blood it may lead to infection.

Suggested remedy: Wash the finger with soap and water and pat dry with a clean paper towel. Clean the cut with non-distilled witch hazel extract or tea tree oil. Apply a natural healing ointment that includes calendula, chickweed, St.-John's-wort, honey, or aloe gel.

Poison Plants and Stinging Nettles

What they are : "Leaves of three, let it be." Two members of the *Rhus* family — poison oak and poison ivy — together with stinging nettles are probably responsible for more human discomfort in the United States than any other plant. These culprits are poisonous to touch and can cause a contact dermatitis in the form of an itchy rash. Weed your garden, pet your dog or cat, and within 48 hours you may be experiencing blisters on your hands.

Suggested remedies for poison ivy: The natural world provides its own remedies for these irritants. Become familiar with sweet fern and jewelweed. They are truly our plant allies against the *Rhus* family.

Cold-water bath. When first exposed, shower in *cold* water. The sooner and longer you shower, the better the chances of minimizing a rash. Soap and warm water are not recommended.

Sweet fern bath. Take a cool bath with the leaves of sweet fern. Native Americans have used the leaves as a wash for poison ivy rash (and in a beverage) since before the time of the Pilgrims. You will often find a sweet fern shrub growing above poison ivy — nature provides if you know where to look.

Vitamin C paste. At the first sign of a poison ivy rash, make a paste of powdered vitamin C mixed with water and apply directly to the affected skin.

Jewelweed. Find and learn to recognize yellow jewelweed. This plant really works. I like to call it nature's antidote for poison ivy. Jewelweed keeps bad company for a good reason, growing in moist ground near poison ivy.

If you are out hiking and think that you have been exposed to poison ivy, pour the water from your canteen over the exposed area. Then, with your handy field guide to medicinal plants, look up jewelweed. If you are lucky in your search, simply crush the stems and leaves and apply directly to the spot. Or if you are camping, chop the stems and cover with water. Boil down half the liquid. You can then use the wilted herb and the fluid to wash away the urushiol oil (the cause of the rash).

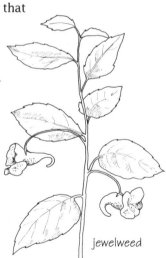

jewelweed

JEWELWEED ICE CUBES

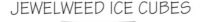

To have the jewelweed remedy ready during the summer at home, here's what you'll need:

Jewelweed leaves and
   stems
Water to cover

To make:

1. Gather the stems and leaves of jewelweed after the dew is off the plants, around 10 to 11 A.M.

2. Cut the plant into 1- to 2-inch pieces. Put the pieces in a plastic bag and flatten with a wooden mallet or rolling pin.

3. Place the crushed plant material in a pot and cover with water.

4. Bring to a boil and simmer until the water is reduced by half and has turned a golden amber color.

5. Cool and strain the plant from the remaining liquid.

6. Pour the liquid into ice cube trays. When frozen, transfer the cubes to a heavy-duty freezer bag and label appropriately.

To use:

The ice cubes will be your magic potion for the summer for all your hiker and gardening friends who suffer the pangs of the poison ivy malady. Soon you will become known as "herb" person when washing with the magic ice cubes cures the rash in a matter of days.

Note: The wilted plant material can be used as a poultice for immediate poison ivy dilemmas. Save the plant material in a covered plastic container in the refrigerator, up to one week.

DON TO THE RESCUE

One of my favorite pastimes is teaching folks how to rid them-
selves of a poison ivy rash. I try to spread the word wherever I go.
Recently, Don, whom I had instructed in the "art of jewelweed," had
the opportunity to help a neighbor. It seems that as the neighbor
was weeding her garden — dressed appropriately in long sleeves,
long pants, and gloves — she unfortunately rubbed her chin.
Within the hour, her chin became red and swollen. Not at all a
pretty sight. And there was a 6 P.M. cocktail party that she was
now sure she could not attend.

Don to the rescue. He grabbed some jewelweed from his garden,
put it in a pot, covered it with water, boiled it down, and applied the
wilted weeds — tied around her head with a strip of muslin — to
her chin. The swelling and redness receded in time for a victorious
entrance to the party. It's great to be a hero!

Suggested remedies for poison oak: On the west coast of the
United States, more people suffer from poison oak. Two plants to
try for treating poison oak rashes are California mugwort and
grindelia, the gum plant. Make a tincture with the flowers of
grindelia and use as a diluted spray on unbroken skin, or make a
wash or poultice with California mugwort and apply to the rash.
Suggested remedies for stinging nettles: The natural antidote for nettle stings is bruised, young, dock leaves. Bandage
the crushed leaves in place; or pound and stir the dock leaves
into cold cream for a healing salve.

Psoriasis

What it is: Psoriasis, a skin problem affecting about 2 percent
of the people in the world, is caused by an overproduction of
epidermal cells. A normal skin cell has a twenty-one- to twenty-
eight-day cycle and then sloughs off. Those with psoriasis turn
over epidermal cells in three or four days, causing the skin
thickness to be five to ten times the norm. Instead of shedding,
these cells build up on the skin, thicken, scale, and crack. Picking at the scales makes them bleed because there is an overgrowth of new blood vessels under the lesions.

Psoriasis appears as patches of thickened, silvery white, scaly skin, often with a red rim. These patches, usually circular or oval in shape, form on the hands, elbows, and knees — parts of the body subjected to the most abrasion. Fingernails and toenails can become rough and pitted. The density of the nail increases, and it may separate from the nail bed.

Suggested remedies: Psoriasis is thought to be hereditary and is not contagious. It can disappear and reappear at certain seasons of the year and is often affected by stress. It is a long-term condition, and at this writing there is no permanent cure. However, there are several natural remedies you can employ that will help you to control outbreaks and soothe the scaly skin patches.

Nutrition. One of the best ways to care for psoriasis is to maintain a diet rich in nutrients beneficial to the skin. Recommended supplements to try daily include granulated soy lecithin, vitamins A, B_6, C, D, and E, and omega-3 oils (a type of essential fatty acid). Fish rich in omega-3s and vitamins A and D are mackerel, lake trout, tuna, salmon, herring, and bluefish. (Ocean fish have more omega-3s than freshwater fish.)

Flaxseed oil. Flaxseed oil is another good source of omega-3s (see recipe on page 154). The recommended dose of flaxseed oil is 1 to 3 tablespoons (15 to 45 ml) per day, to be reduced to 1 to 3 teaspoons (5 to 15 ml) after any improvement is noted. Store this oil in the freezer until it is opened, and then keep it refrigerated. Another alternative is to add flaxseeds to recipes — each tablespoon of flaxseed equals about 1 teaspoon of oil.

Sun and mud. What could be more relaxing than mud baths, sunbathing, and saltwater soaks in the floatable Dead Sea? Israel's Dead Sea vacation area offers sun, spas, and skin treatment centers for folks with psoriasis and other skin disorders.

The Dead Sea — the lowest topographical point on the earth's surface — is full of beneficial trace elements and minerals. Heavy clouds and atmospheric layers filter much of the sunlight reaching sunbathers, eliminating most of the sun's damaging UVB rays. Sunbathers are getting almost pure UVA light and very little UVB and UVC. You are less likely to burn here, but being careful is still prudent. After about twenty-eight days of treatment at the Dead Sea, remissions in psoriasis outbreaks average six to eight months. It works, but this is not a cure. (See page 252 in "Resources" for information on Dead Sea resorts.) If you can't manage a trip to this exotic location, sample some natural skin products that utilize the minerals from this amazing body of water.

OMEGA-3 SHAKE

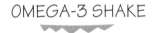

1 tablespoon (15 ml) ground flaxseeds
1 ripe medium banana
3/4 cup (180 ml) blueberries or raspberries, fresh or frozen
1/4 cup (60 ml) low-fat vanilla yogurt
3/4 cup (180 ml) juice of your choice or nonfat soy milk
5 ice cubes or 1/2 cup (125 ml) crushed ice

To make and use:
Toss all the ingredients into a blender and drink or eat with a spoon.

Ring-Finger Rash

What it is: This is an unexplained rash that occurs under a ring due to some irritation. Culprits may be soaps, detergents, waxes, polishes, or cosmetic creams that accumulate under the ring and cause dermatitis. In other cases, minerals found in the rings, such as nickel in costume jewelry and even 9-carat gold, may react with a person's skin and form irritants. Women who are pregnant may experience finger swelling, which causes finger rings to become tighter and traps household chemicals and abrasives beneath. These ingredients rub against the metals in the ring and appear as black smudges on the fingers. **Suggested remedies:** Here are some ways to prevent ring-finger rash.

◆ Clean your rings frequently with a brush inside and out, and periodically soak the rings overnight in ammonia water, using 1 tablespoon (15 ml) ammonia to 2 pints (1 liter) water. Rinse and dry thoroughly.

◆ When your skin chemistry reacts with metals, you may need to upgrade your jewelry and avoid contact with these alloys.

◆ If finger swelling becomes bothersome during pregnancy, remove rings until after the baby arrives.

RING-FINGER SODA PASTE REMEDY

Baking soda, salt, and water make a soothing coating for an irritated ring finger.

1/2 teaspoon (2.5 ml) salt
1/2 teaspoon (2.5 ml) baking soda
Warm water to make a paste

To make:
Make a paste of salt and baking soda with the warm water.

To use:
1. Wash the affected finger with a mild soap and water. Gently pat dry.
2. Spread the paste over the breakout area. Let this paste dry and remain on the finger as long as possible.
3. Repeat once a day till the rash is gone.

Scars and Keloids

What they are: A scar is a mark left in the skin by new connective tissue that replaces tissue injured by a burn, ulcer, incision, or vaccination. Scar tissue is usually stronger and tougher than regular skin. It is formed by special flat, elongated cells called fibroblasts that help construct fibrous tissues in the body.

Keloids are an excessive amount of scar formation caused when the mechanism for producing new connective tissue is out of control, causing an overgrowth of dense, smooth scar tissue. A keloid scar can get worse over time and can also cause pain and itching. Keloids are more common in people with dark skin.

Suggested remedies: To prevent or limit scarring, especially if your skin has a tendency to produce keloid scars, try the following remedies.

St.-John's-wort oil. If pain accompanies a keloid, smooth a small amount of St.-John's-wort oil (see recipe on page 158) over the area.

Vitamin E oil. The liquid contents of vitamin E capsules are extremely helpful in preventing and sometimes even removing scars. Apply the oil directly on the injured tissue.

Vitamin therapy. Regular supplements of vitamin E (400 IU daily) will also help your skin tissue recover from injury with minimal scarring. I prefer a form of natural vitamin E rather than synthetic. Look for "d-alpha tocopherol." The synthetic variety, derived from petrochemicals, is "*di*-alpha tocopherol." If you are prone to keloids, whenever you injure your skin, increase the dose of vitamin E to 1200 IU for a few days and include sufficient zinc in your diet, equal to 15 mg a day for adults. (*Caution:* This large a dose of vitamin E is not recommended for individuals with high blood pressure.) Recent medical findings indicate that zinc is an important trace mineral in healing the skin. Diets rich in whole-grain foods, protein, wheat bran, wheat germ, and brewer's yeast are usually high in zinc.

Lavender essential oil. Applying essential oil of lavender "neat," or undiluted, to injured tissue immediately after injury often prevents excessive scarring. You can also mix a few drops of lavender essential oil with aloe vera gel, apply to the injury, and cover with a sterile gauze pad.

Chickweed oil compress. Chickweed is an old English remedy for healing the skin. Used fresh or in an oil (see recipe below), it has emollient qualities that will help heal cuts and wounds that have begun to crust over or scab, and keep scarring minimal. A chickweed compress is also good for boils, abscesses, and skin irritations such as rashes and eczema.

CHICKWEED OIL

Fresh chickweed, not sprayed with any pesticide
Sunflower seed oil to cover

(Adapted from a recipe by Christopher Hedley, MNIMH.)

To make:
1. Crush the fresh chickweed with a rolling pin in a muslin bag or wrapped in cheesecloth.
2. Fill a jar with the crushed chickweed. Press it firmly to add as much of the herb as possible.
3. Add the oil to cover, with a bit more than needed.
4. Cover with a lid; label and write the date on the jar. Set aside to infuse or steep for two weeks.
5. Strain the oil; pour into clean, dark bottles, cap, and relabel. Store in refrigerator.
To use:
Apply on wounds or skin irritations to facilitate healing.

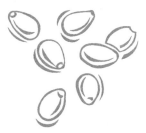

ST.-JOHN'S-WORT OIL

St.-John's-wort *(Hypericum perforatum)* is a sun-loving plant that grows easily in many parts of the world and can be cultivated in your own backyard. The oil made from its flowerheads has both analgesic and antiseptic properties and can be used topically to encourage healing of cuts, scratches, and minor burns and to ease the pain of stiff joints.

Collect just the top two inches of the flowering heads of this plant (some purists collect only the just-opening flowerheads). Shake out the flowers as you pick, to leave any residents in their home locations.

Fresh flowerheads of
St.-John's-wort
Cold-pressed olive oil
to cover

To make:
1. Fill clean, dry, wide-mouthed mason jars to the top, loosely packed, with the fresh herb. Bruise petals with a wooden spoon. Cover with olive oil.
2. Stir with a non-metal utensil (such as a wooden chopstick) to release air bubbles and allow the oil to penetrate the crevices of the flowers. Top off with more oil, seal, and label.
3. Set the sealed jars in direct sunlight, turning every day. Keep an eye out for possible mold that may occur inside the jar, and if it does, wipe it clean with a paper towel. When the oil has turned red (about 3 to 4 weeks), it's ready.
4. First filter it through a fine mesh cheesecloth, and then again through a paper coffee filter. Compost the saturated herb.
5. Pour the filtered red oil into a clean jar. Cover with a double layer of cheesecloth and secure with a rubber band. Let sit for 24 hours to observe. If any sludge or particulate matter settles to the bottom, use a poultry baster to transfer the top oil into another clean jar. Seal, label, and date.

Smelly Hands

What it is: Smelly hands are most often caused by handling fresh fish, garlic, onions, and other pungent foods. Although it's not a major cause for concern, it can be nettlesome in social interactions.

Suggested remedies: Although there's nothing better than a good hard scrub with a deodorizing lovage pad, there are several quick cures for smelly hands:

- *For "fishy" hands:* Rub hands with vinegar or lemon juice to relieve the fishy smell.
- *For pungent garlic hands:* Dry-wash your hands with coffee grounds; the grounds will absorb the garlic smell.
- *For onion hands:* Roll fresh leaves of parsley between your hands; the parsley will neutralize the smell of onion.

Lovage scrub pad. Lovage is a wonderful, celery-like herb with many uses. I use the hollow stems as straws in Bloody Mary drinks and the leaves in chicken soup. But the dried leaves can also be used as a deodorant for hands that retain the smell of onion, garlic, or any other strong-smelling foods. Dry the leaves and keep them in a small cheesecloth or muslin bag. When needed, run the bag under hot tap water and rub the pad over your hands to remove clinging odors. It works wonders.

Splinters

What they are: A splinter is a small foreign fragment that enters the outer layer of the skin, usually on a finger, and causes swelling and irritation. Splinter fragments can be any number of things, from thorns and briars to wood, fiberglass, and metal slivers.

Suggested remedies: Needle-nose tweezers are a good first choice to remove the splinter. When the splinter is in too deep, try one of the kitchen remedies on the following page.

Splinter remedy 1. Wrap a slice of raw bacon over the area of the splinter. Wear this for about 30 minutes, and then try again with your tweezers. The splinter should be easier to remove.

Splinter remedy 2. Before bedtime, coat the finger with olive oil. Then place a piece of adhesive or carpet tape over the splinter. By morning, the splinter should be affixed to the tape or easy to work out of its lodged position.

Warts

What they are: Visually, warts are small, hard, white or pink lumps known as benign skin tumors that are caused by a family of viruses called papillomavirus. The common wart typically appears on the hand but can occur on other parts of the body.

Wart viruses are spread by touch. The virus must come in contact with the skin (even a handshake). If there is a small break or tear in the skin, the virus will have access to deeper, living cells that can then be infected. During the period of damage, the virus will stimulate skin cells to grow and divide, producing the small, visible, warty lesions.

Anyone can have warts. They are most common in teenagers and adults under thirty. Those with suppressed immune systems may be more susceptible.

DISTINGUISHING WARTS AND MOLES

Warts and moles have different appearances. Common warts are hard lumps with a cauliflower-like surface and tiny black flecks that are really the ends of blood vessels. Plantar warts are so named because they appear on the soles of the feet. They are flattened by the pressure of walking. Moles are usually small circles of dark, pigmented skin that can occur anywhere on the body. A mole may be flat or raised and sometimes has hairs growing from it.

Warts are transmitted by viruses. Moles can be present from birth and some may develop during childhood.

Generally, warts are a nuisance but are not dangerous. However, a mole changes in appearance, a physician should check it for the possibility that it has become malignant. It then may need to be removed.

Suggested remedies: Fifty percent of all warts will disappear without treatment. Seventy percent that are surgically or chemically removed stay away. The rest are a continual nuisance. Scratching and picking at warts spreads them by bringing existing viruses to the surface; scratching also stimulates the mother wart to enlarge and thicken. If you suffer from warts, try applications of any of the following natural remedies.

Greater celandine juice: Put a few drops of the fresh, orange-yellow juice from the stem of the greater celandine plant directly on the wart. Allow the juice to dry and remain on the spot for as long as possible. Repeat daily until the wart begins to disappear. It can be a slow process but it is usually successful. Discontinue if there is any unusual burning sensation. *Caution:* Do not use this herb if you are pregnant. Don't use celandine on the face or on large clusters of warts.

Willow bark: James Duke, Ph.D., author of *The Green Pharmacy,* suggests taping a small, moistened piece of the inner bark of a willow tree to the wart. Apply a new piece of inner bark daily for five to seven days.

KISS THE PRINCE

Shortly before her wedding, my friend's daughter, Karen, came to me with the problem of warts. At that time, I had not used celandine as a treatment but had heard of its long folk usage. Karen and her fiancé had purchased a home and invited me to visit. Their house faced on a small wooded lot and the previous owners had been away for a while. As I walked up the front steps, there, growing in the cracks, was *Chelidonium majus* itself. I began to think that there is no such thing as a coincidence.

Karen was willing to try an experiment with the caveat that if there was any discomfort, she would immediately rinse off the liquid. Every day, she dabbed the brightly colored celandine stem juice on her warts. The warts began to shrink and were completely gone in time for the wedding. This trial does not a research study make, but it is folk history repeating itself.

GARLIC OIL

If neither willow bark nor celandine is readily available, a traditional remedy you can use on warts is garlic oil.

1 bulb fresh garlic, peeled, divided into cloves, and chopped

Olive oil to cover

To make:

1. Refrigerate the chopped garlic cloves in the oil overnight.

2. Strain out the cloves and pour the oil into a small bottle, label, and date.

3. Store in the refrigerator.

To use:

Dab this oil on the wart with a cotton swab or on an adhesive bandage applied to the wart.

HEALING IS BELIEF

My grandmother, born and brought up in Russia, believed in and used many folk remedies. Bubbie Sophie would rub a copper penny on a grandchild's finger wart, say a prayer, and see the wart disappear in short order. What stimulated the immune system to attack and destroy the wart? Was copper the cure? Perhaps it was only the belief that the wart would disappear. There is still much we do not know about the relationship between psychological stimuli and our immune systems.

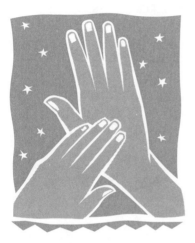

Flexibility and
Movement:
Caring for the
Joints of the
Fingers, Thumbs,
Wrists, and Elbows

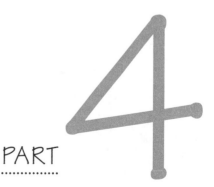

PART

4

CHAPTER 9
Exercises and Remedies for Injured Joints

Fingers were made before forks and hands before knives.
— Jonathan Swift

Whether swinging a tennis racket, playing the guitar, folding an omelet, or typing on a keyboard, human fingers, wrists, arms, and elbows are designed for movement. The undercover structures that allow this ingenious machinery to function include a bony skeleton, tendons, muscles, lubricating membranes, and pliable skin. To allow the movement of which we are capable, each of these structures meets and functions cooperatively at our joints.

WHAT IS A JOINT?

A joint is the site where two bones meet and are bound together. The structure of a joint, as well as the way its constituent parts work together, determine the ways in which it can move. A synovial joint is enclosed within a joint capsule, a layer of fibrous tissue with an inner lining called the synovial membrane. There are six parts to each synovial joint:

Cartilage. The ends of each bone are cushioned and protected by a layer of rubbery connective tissue called cartilage. Feel the central spine of your nose or above the lobe of your ear for a sense of the structure of cartilage. Cartilage has no nerve endings, so cartilage-coated surfaces can make contact without causing pain (or any other sensation). The pain associated with osteoarthritis often results from the wearing away of this cartilage coating in the joints.

Muscles. These elastic tissues stretch and contract to move bones and move us.

Ligaments. Ligaments are short, fibrous bands of tissue that tie bone to bone and enclose the joint capsule.

Tendons. Muscles are attached to the bones by the fibrous tendon cords. You can observe the movement of tendons on the back of your hand.

Synovial membrane. Surrounding each joint site is a synovial sac — a smooth, thin layer of tissue filled with a transparent, egg-white-like fluid. This fluid coats and protects the inner surface of the ligaments and the cartilage that caps the end of the bones.

Bursae. Next to the joint capsule are smaller, fluid-filled lubricating sacs called bursae. Bursae are not always considered components of the joint, but they do serve several important functions: to reduce friction between tendons and ligaments and between tendons and bones; to maintain joint mobility; and to allow the structures to glide freely in relation to each other. Excessive use or injury to a joint can swell these sacs and cause bursitis. Tennis elbow is a form of bursitis inflammation.

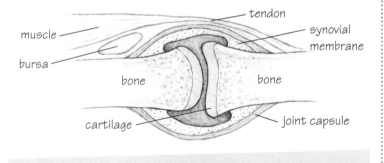

DOUBLE-JOINTED?

Yes and no! This colloquial term refers to someone who has unusually flexible joints with an exceptional degree of freedom of motion. In elementary school, I recall a boy who could bend his thumb backward until it touched his wrist! Perhaps you have stood in awe of the "pretzel-man" in the circus who could wrap his legs around his ears. An amazing feat (no pun intended) but not really a double joint.

TYPES OF JOINTS

There are three types of synovial joints in the hands and arms: hinge joints, saddle joints, and pivot joints.

Hinge joints act like the hinge on a screen door and allow movement in only one direction. Examples of this type of joint are the fingers, knuckles, and elbow.

Saddle joints permit movement in two planes or directions. A saddle joint connects the base of the thumb to the hand, giving us a strong, firm, flexible grip.

A pivot joint allows rotation of a bone relative to another bone, permitting the wrist its twisting, pivot-like movement.

WHAT MAKES A KNUCKLE CRACK?

Believe it or not, the answer to this simple question was a mystery until 1971. Then scientists in Britain traced the popping noise to the bursting of gas bubbles in the synovial fluid inside the joint capsule. The bubbles form when a joint is stretched and pressure on the synovial fluid is reduced. Eventually the bubbles pop, just as you see liquid soap bubbles burst in the air. Inside the joints, however, the gas from the bubble cannot break out, and it must gradually return to the fluid. It takes about 15 minutes for the gas to return to the fluid. A noisy knuckle-cracker will have to wait a quarter of an hour before beginning another performance.

PROTECTING YOUR JOINTS

In time, all of us are affected by the stiffness and aches resulting from overuse of our joints. Here are a few suggestions for protecting the joints in your hands and wrists. If you put your mind to it, I'm sure you will be able to think of several more ideas.

◆ Let your larger joints do the work in place of smaller joints. For instance, carry hangers from the cleaners over your arm and save those finger joints, and instead of carrying a heavy bag or briefcase in your hand, switch to a shoulder strap that transfers the weight to a larger joint.

- ◆ Avoid favoring a particular finger or position with the hands.
- ◆ Use a food processor or slicing machine instead of a knife (less force on the fingers).
- ◆ Use a jar opener to open jars to avoid extra force on the hands and finger joints.
- ◆ Use foam padding around a pen or a pencil, a fork, toothbrush, or razor for less joint stress in these everyday tasks (see "Resources" for Grab On padding products).
- ◆ Take a break from repetitive tasks, such as computer work, machinery, and bread baking. Gently stretch your hands and arms several times a day. (For stretching exercises, see pages 168 and 169.)
- ◆ When gardening or doing yardwork, use the innovative "enabling tools" that are designed to remove stress points from fingers and wrists.

WRITER'S CRAMP

In the *Practical Home Physician* of 1888 under "Diseases of the Nervous System," there is a listing for "writer's cramp." The disorder is described as "a form of paralysis usually limited to certain muscles of the hand . . . common among those whose occupation compels them to hold the pen many hours a day . . . . Writers . . . tailors, and sewing girls who are compelled to use the same muscles constantly for many hours daily, are often similarly affected."

Signs of writer's cramp are weakened power in the movement of the finger and thumb and, in some cases, contraction of the muscles controlling the fingers, so that the thumb and fingers cannot be moved or move only irregularly. Treatment includes rest and massage of the affected parts.

With the advent of computer technology, it seems we have replaced this ailment with a new one, carpal tunnel syndrome, which often affects those who must sit at computer terminals for hours every day. We just can't seem to get ahead!

STRENGTHENING YOUR JOINTS

Here are some great finger, hand, and wrist exercises for flexibility, strength, and preventive care that you can do anywhere. This time, no pain equals gain!

Rhythmic Finger Moves to Music

This series of exercises is designed and shared by international fitness consultant Barbara Barsham. She claims that a daily dose of these spirited movements will keep your fingers limber and able to do all the finger things you've gotten used to doing!

This is a good warm-up exercise to improve finger coordination and your mood. No special equipment is needed (except you might want to locate a tape or CD of lively piano music).

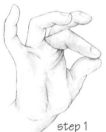

step 1

Step 1: Thumb-tap. One by one, tap the fingerpads of each finger to the thumb: index to thumb, middle to thumb, ring finger to thumb, and pinkie to thumb, counting 1-2-3-4; then reverse, pinkie to thumb, ring to thumb, middle to thumb, and index to thumb, 4-3-2-1. This should be easy and cause no discomfort. Ten times on each hand is a good goal to work toward. Then try both hands at the same time.

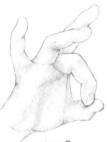

step 2

Step 2: Thumb-flick. Follow the same procedure, but this time flick each nail off the thumb as if flicking off a piece of lint.

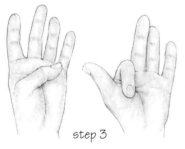

step 3

Step 3: Finger-palm. With fingers held as straight as possible, touch each one, beginning with your thumb, to your palm in turn, and then reverse and do it again, beginning with your pinkie.

Step 4: Piano scales. Pretend there's a piano above your head, almost out of reach. Stretch both hands up above your head and play the scales on the imaginary piano: C, D, E, F, G — G, F, E, D, C. (For those of you who don't know the scales, pretend you're striking adjacent keys on a piano, one key per finger.) Do this several times. Then bring your hands down to waist level and repeat the procedure, forward and backward.

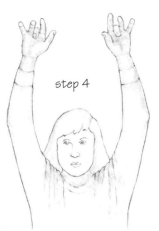

step 4

Last, form your fingers into bent claws and try to play up and down the piano scales again.

Step 5: Finger stretch. With your hands at your sides and your thumbs pointing toward your body, spread your thumbs and fingers as far as they can go and stretch. Hold for a count of five. Then close them to a fist and hold for a count of ten. Relax. Repeat ten times.

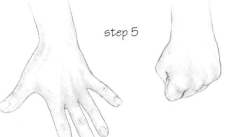

step 5

The hand grip of a seventy-five-year-old is normally only three-fourths as strong as that of a thirty-year-old. Regular exercise will slow the decline.

Is this what they mean when they say, "You're losing your grip"?

Chinese Exercise Balls

Chinese exercise balls are perfectly weighted, hollow, polished chrome or glazed balls that fit comfortably, two at a time, into your palm. They emit a wonderful, delicate chime as they move. The balls are available in different sizes to accommodate large and small hands. To judge the best size for you, hold two balls in a hand. Your fingers should be able to clasp and cover both balls comfortably. You'll find these balls in Oriental gift shops, and they are often available in health food stores.

It's believed that regularly rotating Chinese exercise balls in the palm of each hand not only stimulates the fingers but also taps acupuncture points, improving the circulation of vital energy throughout the body. Use these exercise balls to combat numbness of the fingers and trembling hands, as well as arthritis in the fingers and wrist. Manufacturers of these balls claim that using them "will keep the muscles nimble, the bones strong, the mind sober, the memory intact, relieve fatigue, prevent and cure hypertension, drown your worries, and prolong life." The balls can also be very effective for relaxation and meditation once you get the hang of it. All ages will find them a fun and worthwhile habit.

ROARING DRAGON AND SINGING PHOENIX

Ancient Chinese mandarins believed that palm-size exercise balls induced well-being of the body and serenity of spirit. First hand-forged more than eight hundred years ago by a blacksmith in Baoding, China, these hollow, iron balls were fashioned with a unique metal soundboard inside. There were two special sounds — one pitched high and the other pitched low — symbolizing yin and yang, and the tones of the roar of the dragon and the song of the phoenix that lived on and roamed the grounds of the fabled Yan-Chi Palace. An emperor during the Ming dynasty was so pleased with these balls that he declared them one of the "three treasures" of Baoding.

This exercise calls into motion all the joints of the hand and elbow as well as the muscles of the forearm. It warms the hands and stimulates circulation in the fingers and in the palms of your hands. Begin with your dominant hand and then switch. Start over a table so you won't have to run after the balls as they fall.

After you become comfortable with the routine, try doing this exercise daily, while reading or watching television. If you really get into this, you might increase to three or four balls.

Step 1: Put two balls in the palm of your hand. Rotate the balls in a clockwise direction using your thumb and all the fingers as guides. Try to work up a regular, smooth rhythm over several minutes before switching to the reverse direction.

Step 2: Reverse direction and go counterclockwise. This is a larger challenge for the fingers and brain.

SPRAINS

A sprain is the twisting or wrenching of a joint with partial damage to its attachments but without dislocating bones. Depending on the degree of injury to the ligaments, the pain can be greater than having a broken bone and is especially intensified by movement. The signs of a sprain are rapid swelling, the feeling of heat, and difficulty in movement of the joint.

For immediate care of sprains, remember this word: *I-C-E.* It stands for **I**ce, **C**ompression, and **E**levation. To keep down the swelling and pain of a sprain, you should ice (if you have a bag of frozen peas or corn in the freezer, that will work just as well as an icepack), wrap, and elevate the injured joint as soon as possible! You can then try the herbal compress on page 172.

"SPRAINS A DRAIN" COMPRESS

This is a soothing herbal remedy that is very effective on a sprain. Both St.-John's-wort oil and arnica extract are worth having in your home or travel first-aid kit. First apply ice to the sprained finger, wrist, or elbow to minimize swelling, and then wrap in this compress.

1–4 teaspoons (5–20 ml) arnica extract
2 cups (500 ml) hot water
Burdock leaves or green cabbage leaves
2 cups (500 ml) boiling water
St.-John's-wort oil (see recipe on page 158)

To make:

1. Prepare a solution of arnica and hot water. A standard infusion is 1 to 4 teaspoons (5 to 20 ml) extract in 2 cups (500 ml) hot water.

2. Pound the fresh burdock or cabbage leaves, and then immerse them in boiling water for 2 minutes. Drain leaves on paper towels.

To use:

1. Coat the skin of the sprained area with St.-John's-wort oil.

2. Dip a soft, thin towel in the warm arnica wash. Squeeze out excess liquid and apply the towel to the sprain.

3. Cover with the warm wilted burdock or green cabbage leaves.

4. Wrap with wide gauze to hold the compress in place. Elevate the injured joint. Repeat twice a day until the swelling is gone.

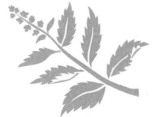

CARPAL TUNNEL SYNDROME

Carpal tunnel syndrome is an injury associated with repetitive motion. If you spend long hours at your computer terminal, if you are a musician or a factory worker with a high-force, highly repetitious task, or if you face any other type of repetitive hand-wrist movement, you may be susceptible to this ailment. The injury usually begins with numbness and tingling or burning in the fingers. It can progress to pain and decreased strength and coordination of the hands and a limited range of motion in the forearm and upper arm. Unfortunately, sometimes this pain travels to the armpit, shoulder, and neck and, in very serious cases, may require surgery.

Anatomy of the Carpal Tunnel

The carpal tunnel is created by the bones of the wrist, which are laid out in a contour that resembles a shallow basin. There is a narrow opening in the palm side of the wrist made up of eight wrist or carpal bones. Three walls of the "tunnel" consist of these carpal bones, while the fourth "wall" is formed by the transverse carpal ligament, a strap of tough ligament.

The carpal tunnel is a very crowded section. Nine tendons (controlling movement of the hand and fingers) and the median nerve (assisting movement and sensation in the hand and fingers) pass through the carpal tunnel under the transverse carpal ligament. As the fingers move and repeat a movement again and again, the area inside the ligament can become irritated, causing the tendons to swell and to squeeze the median nerve. Pressure on the median nerve can cause symptoms of discomfort in the fingers, hand, and elbow. These symptoms may include the sensation of numbness (often most noticeable at night), tingling, burning, cold, pain, and stiffness, or physical problems with grip strength and thumb weakness, depending on how intense the pressure on the nerve is.

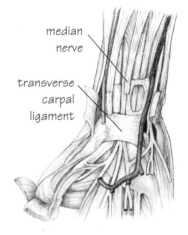

median nerve

transverse carpal ligament

anatomy of the carpal tunnel

Testing for Carpal Tunnel Syndrome

If you are concerned that you might have carpal tunnel syndrome, there are a couple of simple tests you can perform at home. However, it is important to get an appropriate diagnosis before treating carpal tunnel syndrome, so be sure to see a knowledgeable healthcare professional. More extensive tests include magnetic resonance imaging (MRI), computerized tomography (CT) scans, and electromyography (EMG).

Phalen's test: Place your elbows on a surface and allow your hands to relax to a 90-degree angle at the wrists. Or gently place the backs of the hands together with no force, and hold this position for 1 minute. If you feel any numbness, tingling, or pain in your thumb, index finger, or ring finger, the test is positive. (Phalen's test is correct in diagnosing carpal tunnel syndrome about 75 to 80 percent of the time.)

Tinel's test: This is also known as the median nerve percussion test. Place your hand palm-side up on a table. Tap the area over the median nerve with the index finger of the opposite hand. If you feel tingling or numbness, the test is positive. (Tinel's test is correct in diagnosing carpal tunnel syndrome about 65 percent of the time.)

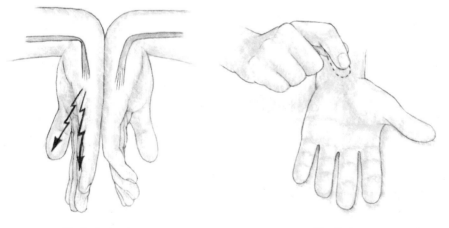

Phalen's test   Tinel's test

Natural Care for Carpal Tunnel

Specially designed soft, slow, gentle stretching exercises can bring relief to those with carpal tunnel or other repetitive strain injuries. Sharon Butler, in *Conquering Carpal Tunnel,* talks about the concept of a "stretch point." This is the first hint of a stretch, a slight resistance to the movement. It will appear at the beginning of the stretch and fade as the tissue releases. This loosening is the beginning of change and of healing. She suggests that it helps to close your eyes when practicing stretching exercises. For each of these exercises, start with one set of ten repetitions and build up to three sets of ten each time.

DADDY LONGLEGS HANDSTAND

You can do this exercise seated at a table or walking your hand up a wall.

Step 1: Begin with the palm and fingers flat on the surface.

Step 2: Put gentle pressure on the thumb and little finger and raise the hand up on all the fingers, like a daddy longlegs. Hold and count to 5, and slowly slide back down. Repeat with each hand five times as long as there is no pain.

step 1

step 2

WINDSHIELD WIPER HANDS

This is an easy wrist stretch. It may be a windshield wiper experience, but hopefully you will have a sunny day!

Step 1: You are seated and resting one arm on a table. Move one hand as a windshield wiper would function, side-to-side, toward the thumb and then away from the thumb. Do 10 repetitions in each direction. Repeat with the other hand.

Step 2: Place both forearms on the table. Lift at the wrist and bring index fingers together and then apart. Continue inward, outward.

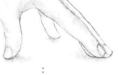

step 2

GENTLE WRIST FLEX

Step 1: Extend one arm in front of you with palm and fingers facing up.

Step 2: Take the other hand and place it sideways across the outstretched palm, as in reaching for a handshake.

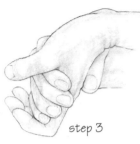

step 3

Step 3: Press gently against the palm and the fingers for a mild extension. Repeat on the opposite side. This is an easy and important stretch to do when you are spending a lot of time in front of a computer.

Step 4: For this slightly more vigorous stretch, hang your hand, palm-side down, over a shelf, table, or armchair. Use your other hand to bend it down as far as comfortably possible. Repeat with the opposite hand.

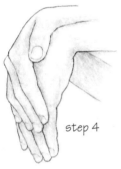

step 4

WISHING POSE PRESS

Step 1: Put both hands together, palms touching and fingers interlaced.
Step 2: Pressing the palms, push the right hand backward with the force of the left.
Step 3: Reverse, pushing the left hand backward with the strength of the right. The pressure should emanate from the palms, not the fingers. Bend just till the feeling of discomfort.

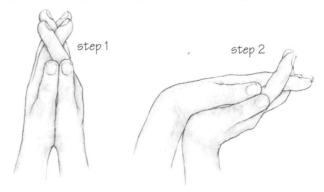

step 1   step 2

WINGS WRIST STRETCH

Step 1: Place your palms together in front of your chest, fingers pointed up.

Step 2: Keeping palms together, slowly raise elbows up as far as possible without discomfort. Release. Repeat slowly.

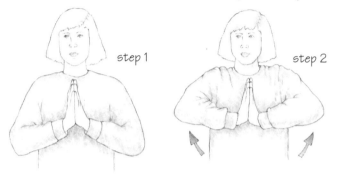

step 1

step 2

FAR EAST WRIST STRETCH

A gentle, isometric stretch for wrists and fingers, this exercise provides elements of stretching, flexing, and range of motion.

Step 1: Place your hands together with the fingers pointing upward in a prayer position or in a hand position you might see as a welcoming greeting if you visited the Far East.

Step 2: Extend your thumbs in a right angle from your fingers. Keep your fingers together.

Step 3: Now, open and spread your fingers while slowly pushing fingertip against fingertip. Extend your fingers as far apart as you can and still be comfortable. It will look as if you are forming a miniature temple with your hands. Hold as if you were doing isometrics for a count of ten. Relax back to a closed-fingers-and-thumb position.

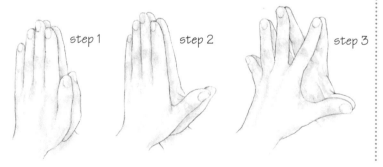

step 1

step 2

step 3

GINGER WARMING COMPRESS

Ginger is a natural circulatory stimulant and an anti-inflammatory herb that has been used for centuries, both internally and externally, in folk medicine. This warming compress will help to relieve pain.

1 piece fresh gingerroot
2 quarts (2 liters) boiling water
St.-John's-wort oil (optional; see recipe on page 158)

To make:

1. Grate fresh gingerroot and tie it in cheesecloth.
2. Put the ginger into the boiling water. Reduce heat and simmer for 30 minutes.
3. Cool to a warm but comfortable temperature.

To use:

1. If the skin on your hands and wrists is very sensitive, apply a thin layer of St.-John's-wort oil to the area around the wrist before you apply the compress.
2. Remove the cheesecloth with the gingerroot. Dip a clean hand towel into the ginger water. Wring out the excess liquid and apply the comfortably warm cloth to the tender wrist area.
3. Cover with a dry towel to insulate the heat.
4. Rewarm every 5 minutes, as desired.

DUPUYTREN'S CONTRACTURE

Named after a celebrated French surgeon, Baron Guillaume Dupuytren (1775–1835), this disease, pronounced du'-pwe-trahnz, causes a progressive inability to straighten both the ring and little fingers. Ultimately, it results in these two fingers becoming permanently fixed in a flexed position. It is thought to be caused by an increase in the *fascia* (bands of short, thick, fibrous tissue) beneath the skin on the palm side of the hand. This thickening causes contraction or tightening of the tendon sheaths of the fourth and fifth fingers.

Genetics seems to play a role in determining the population suffering from this syndrome. It was once thought that those most affected were of Nordic descent (especially young adult men or, sometimes, women after midlife), but there were also those in vocations that required their hands to be in a constantly flexed position, such as boatmen, shoemakers, and carpenters, who suffered from the disease. And today, Dupuytren's contracture is also observed in those with diabetes and epilepsy as well as those who overindulge in alcohol and smoking.

To date, treatment has generally been limited to surgery to relieve the contracture. However, it has been noted that individuals with Dupuytren's contracture tend to have excess lipids (fatty substances) in their blood and a high serum cholesterol. New strategies are being directed toward prevention, and may include some of the same protocols as for treating high cholesterol.

There are some simple, natural approaches to treating Dupuytren's contracture that, although they are not a cure for the disease, may ease or prolong the onset of its symptoms. To potentially save a hand, a lifestyle change is worth a try. Begin by reducing the fat and cholesterol in your diet, especially animal fat. If you smoke, stop, and limit your alcohol intake to extreme moderation. Increase the amount of exercise you get. Also increase the amount of garlic, oats, and bran in your diet, as they have been shown to significantly reduce serum cholesterol and triglyceride levels.

If you suffer from this syndrome, arrange with a healthcare provider to check your lipid levels, and ask about new treatment research.

TRIGGER FINGER

A trigger finger results from obstruction of the *flexor tendon* as a result of repetitive use or trauma to a finger or thumb, which may cause localized swelling of the tendon. This swelling, and/or the knot-like callous of scar tissue that it may cause as the swollen tendon constantly rubs internally, causes the finger to become stuck as it moves through the space of the *A-1 pulley.* The A-1 pulley is a structure that holds a tendon close to the bone and normally helps to increase the efficiency of the flexor tendon.

Trigger finger causes jerky movements of the finger, and may even cause the finger to become locked in a flexed position. It commonly affects the ring and middle fingers, and is four times more prevalent in women than men. In severe cases, trigger finger may require surgical repair.

Natural treatment focuses on resting the finger from its habitual use. Use cushiony foam grips on pens, pencils, and tools, and at night support the finger with a custom-molded splint on the top finger joint, nearest the fingernail. Try dry brushing to stimulate circulation (see page 108) and daily hand soaks (see recipe below) to reduce swelling. To speed healing and reduce scar tissue formation, supplement your diet with vitamin E and zinc.

DEAD SEA SALT HAND BATH

This is a helpful hand soak suitable for all types of overuse injuries, including trigger finger. Dead Sea salts are warming and relaxing.

2 quarts (2 liters) boiling water

1 teaspoon (5 ml) Dead Sea bath salt

2/3 teaspoon (3 ml) Epsom salts

1/3 teaspoon (2 ml) baking soda

2 drops essential oil of your choice: lavender, juniper, cypress, rosemary, or grapefruit

To make:

1. Pour the boiling water into a large, hand-size ceramic or glass bowl.

2. Add the sea salt, Epsom salts, and baking soda. Stir to dissolve. Stir in the essential oil.

To use:

When the water has cooled to a comfortable temperature, soak the affected hand until the water has cooled (about 5 to 10 minutes). If treating a finger, be sure to soak the entire hand, not just the finger.

TENNIS ELBOW AND GOLFER'S ELBOW

These classic elbow injuries are basically a result of overuse. Anyone who uses one arm in repetitive tasks is subject to this discomfort — even children who play video games for hours on end.

Tennis Elbow

Tennis elbow is the result of repetitive wrist extension (straightening or bending back), as used with a tennis player's backhand swing. The muscles that control wrist extension originate on the outside, upper surface of the elbow joint. With overuse, the tendons and ligaments at that tendon-bone juncture begin to micro-tear and swell. Finger and elbow extensors can be affected, and the elbow and forearm become painful to use.

Golfer's Elbow

This repetitive motion injury involves the muscles that control wrist flexion (bending in), as used for a golfer's swing. These muscles originate at the inner, upper surface of the elbow joint. As with tennis elbow, overuse initiates micro-tears and inflammation of the tendons and ligaments at this tendon-bone juncture, and the area becomes painful to use.

Natural Care for Tennis and Golfer's Elbow

If you believe you have tennis or golfer's elbow, you should first have the condition diagnosed by a healthcare professional to determine the extent of your injury and to ensure that it isn't something even more serious. Once diagnosed, any of the following tips will encourage a speedy recovery.

- ◆ **Rest.** The most important step in relieving this type of injury is to stop the repetitive behavior that is causing the injury and to rest the hurt elbow.
- ◆ **Ice.** Apply ice packs (or a bag of frozen corn or peas) to help reduce the inflammation. Apply for 10 to 15 minutes several times a day.

press here
on the non-
injured arm

◆ **Support.** A forearm brace may also be effective in relieving the pain in the elbow and forearm. Be careful not to cut off circulation to your hand — the brace should fit comfortably.

◆ **Point stimulation.** Pressure point stimulation may help to alleviate pain and release muscular tension. For golfer's or tennis elbow, there are two pressure points on the *opposite* arm from the injury.

Step 1: With the fingers extended in a straight position, press the outside edge of the knuckle of your little finger on the *noninjured arm*. Hold for a few seconds, then rest and repeat several times.

Step 2: Now find the exact point of greatest pain on the arm with the injury and press the corresponding point on the *opposite arm*. Same procedure — hold for a count of three and repeat.

PRESSURE POINT NOTE

If you can't find the exact tender spot on the injured elbow, poke around. Pressure points tend to be a bit more sensitive than the surrounding area. Your tools are the tips of your index or middle finger, or both, side by side. Sometimes the thumb is a better choice.

On the opposite arm, a few seconds of pressure applied to that same spot, repeated several times, is all that is needed to help relieve pain. Push gently until you feel slight discomfort.

Strengthening Exercises for the Elbows

Strengthening your elbow joints will help prevent overuse injuries such as tennis and golfer's elbow from plaguing you. Do these exercises only after the pain has subsided. Check with your healthcare provider before attempting these steps.

Forward arm extension: Bend your arm at the elbow with your forearm and palm pointing upward. Support the elbow with the fingers of the other hand. Gently straighten the bent elbow with palm outstretched in front of you, and carefully press the bones in the elbow into the joint. This helps to realign the elbow joint. If possible, repeat three times on each side.

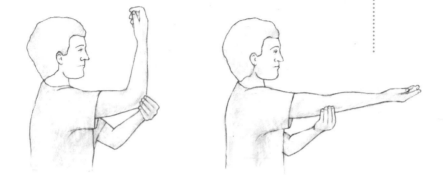

Biceps bulge: Obtain a wide stretch band, about 12 to 18 inches (30 to 45 cm) long when fully extended. (You can find them through rehabilitation centers or from a physical therapist. There are different tensions available in these bands. Begin with the least resistance.) With your arms in front of you, place the band around both of your forearms. Try to bend one elbow up toward your chest as the other elbow straightens out away from the chest. Hold this position for 10 seconds. Alternate left to right. Do not work against pain.

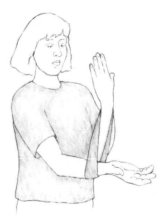

Wrist extension: Rest your arm on a table with your hand, palm-side down, hanging over the edge. Raise your hand in a slow wave, up and down, going to the extremes of your flexibility. Be sure that you are moving only your hand and not your forearm. Start with 5 repetitions and work up to 10, practicing at least once a day. Use this as a daily warmup exercise before any hand activities. Once you are pain-free, you may want to add resistance.

CHAPTER 10
Arthritic Hands

If I have learned one thing, then, it is to believe — not in the impossible but in the possibility of the impossible. Man's ingenuity surprises us with new miracles time and again, whether dreamed about and then proved through many years of hard work in laboratories, or discovered by mere chance.
— Walter Sorrell, *The Story of the Human Hand*

More than forty million Americans — about one in every seven people — suffer from one kind of arthritis or another. There are more than one hundred forms of this disease that somehow cause problems with joints in the body. Each person with arthritis is different. There is no one treatment that is right for everyone. However, all arthritis can be helped in some way.

OSTEOARTHRITIS

Osteoarthritis, the most common form of arthritis, is seen primarily in those over the age of fifty. However, degenerative changes in the joints can occur even in our twenties. This joint disease involves the breakdown of cartilage, the elastic substance that covers and protects the ends of bones in a joint. It can be caused by normal wear and tear or overuse, or it can be inherited.

Cartilage, a form of connective tissue, does not have its own blood supply and receives its oxygen and nutrition from the surrounding joint fluid. When we move a joint, the pressure squeezes fluid and waste products out of the cartilage. As the pressure is relieved, synovial fluid and nutrients seep back into this connective tissue. Over time and use, the cartilage may fray or wear away. The bony surfaces in the joint will then begin to grate against each other. The bone, unlike cartilage, has nerve endings, so the grating causes pain. This doesn't seem fair — our joints should last a lifetime.

Osteoarthritis in the hands most often affects the joints nearest the fingernails and the joint at the base of the thumb. The mildest form causes Heberden's nodes — knobby, bony enlargements of the finger joints — over a period of years. More severe forms can impede movement of the fingers, thumb, and hand.

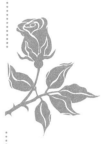

REPAIRING JOINTS WITH GLUCOSAMINE SULFATE

A nutritional supplement called glucosamine sulfate, a naturally occurring substance in joint structures, may help the body repair damaged joints. The body naturally uses glucosamine to stimulate the manufacture of cartilage components involved in the strength and integrity of joint structures. As we age, it seems we lose some of this internal capability to manufacture levels of glucosamine sufficient to maintain joint structure.

Many studies in Europe and in the United States have examined the effects of glucosamine sulfate supplements for those with osteoarthritis.

In general, the test results were positive — the glucosamine was well absorbed and tolerated by the body and, once metabolized, seemed to rest in joint cartilage. Relief has not been instantaneous but many participants with osteoarthritis reported improvement in pain, swelling, and range of joint motion within four to six weeks. It is still not known whether this supplement will have the long-term capacity to encourage strong, durable cartilage in joints.

The dosage suggested by these studies is one 500 mg capsule of glucosamine sulfate three times a day with meals. A possible side effect is heartburn or gas. As a nutritional supplement, this substance is not regulated by the Food and Drug Administration. Ask your healthcare provider for the most current information about glucosamine, and discuss whether this supplement is right for you.

Heberden's Finger Nodes

What it is: The bony knobs that form on the sides of the end, or distal, joints of the fingers are called Heberden's nodes after the British doctor, William Heberden (1710–1801), who first described them. In the affected joints, the cartilage gradually deteriorates, followed by the formation of bony spurs in the joint margins. Finger deformity and limitation of motion results. Range-of-motion exercises for the fingers and wrist, such as playing the piano and knitting, may help keep your joints limber.

Suggested remedies: There is no immediate solution for getting rid of the unsightly finger knobs. Early treatment with glucosamine sulfate (see box on page 185) may reduce some of the damage.

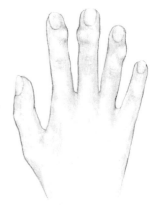

Heberden's nodes

▼▼▼▼▼ SAINT HILDEGARD OF BINGEN'S SALVE

A salve recipe of the Middle Ages, originally prepared by Hildegard von Bingen — a medieval abbess, mystic, and herbalist who was a pioneer in science and authored several works on medicine and natural history — is still being produced today in Munich, Germany (see listing for Max Emanuel Apotheke in "Resources") under the name *Wermutsalbe* (vermouth salve). A member of the New England Unit of the Herb Society sent me a sample. In her words, "When you have stiff hands from arthritis or whatever, this cream gives you movement back." It includes:

◆ 16 grams *Hirschfett* (stag fat)
◆ 6 grams *Hirschmark* (stag marrow)
◆ 8 grams olive oil
◆ 10 grams *frisches Wermutkraut* (fresh vermouth weed)

▲▲▲▲

RHEUMATOID ARTHRITIS

Rheumatoid arthritis is a more complicated, destructive disease than is osteoarthritis. It is chronic, systemic, and typically affects about one-half of 1 percent of the population in the United States, or about one million people. Women are affected three times as frequently as men, and the disease typically rears its ugly head around midlife, although there are exceptions.

Rheumatoid arthritis causes the lining and lubricating membrane of the joints — the synovial membrane — to become inflamed. The cells in this membrane begin to divide and grow, bringing inflammatory cells and releasing enzymes into the joint space. The joint becomes swollen, puffy, and warm. An overabundance of fluid in the inflamed membrane causes swelling, body aches, fatigue, morning stiffness, restriction of joint movement, and, later, destruction of the bone. It can be very painful.

The most commonly affected joints are those of the wrists and knuckles, feet and ankles, and knees. This kind of arthritis may appear symmetrically on both sides of the body, that is, at the base of the fingers on both hands, the knuckles, and the wrists. Lumps the size of a pea may form beneath the skin. These nodules are most commonly located near the elbow. These are inflammations of small blood vessels and will appear and disappear. Blood tests can help in the diagnosis of rheumatoid arthritis. It is prudent to form a good relationship with a specialist in arthritis — a rheumatologist — since early intervention is the best way to proceed with this condition.

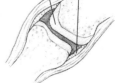

synovial membrane
cartilage

normal joint

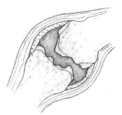

joint afflicted
with osteoarthritis

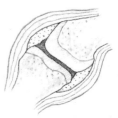

joint afflicted with
rheumatoid arthritis

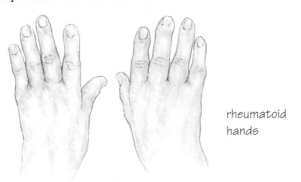

rheumatoid
hands

Tips for Living with Rheumatoid Arthritis

Until a total solution to this problem is presented, the most important goal is to try to maintain functions in the activities of daily living. That means to reduce inflammation and preserve joint movements, range of motion, and physical strength. When exercising other parts of the body, consider the stress imposed on your hands and modify the activity, if possible. Below are some tips for maintaining strength and flexibility in hands with rheumatoid arthritis. If you have severe involvement or hand deformity, consult a hand therapist to help you plan a program.

Exercise. Regular exercise to build muscle tone and increase energy is essential. Exercising a hot, inflamed joint is not encouraged, but it is worthwhile to try to move the hand through its whole range of motion at least twice a day. (See joint exercises for the hand on pages 168–177.)

Heat. Perform hand exercises in a basin of warm water to lessen discomfort. Heat eases pain and reduces muscle spasms. (See also Caramel Cubes on page 191 and Paraffin Hand Bath on page 192.)

Stretch. The general rule for stretching exercises is to move the joint as far as it will comfortably go and then coax it just a little farther, just past the point of first pain. Be gentle and work for a sustained stretch; do not "bounce." (See exercises for boggy finger on pages 189 and 190.)

Omega-3. Nutritional researchers have found that omega-3 oils (a type of essential fatty acid) help to reduce the inflammatory process that characterizes rheumatoid arthritis. The recommended intake of omega-3s is 0.8 to 1.8 grams per day (and more is not better) in a fish-oil supplement. A diet containing bony fish two or three times a week should provide a balanced level of omega-3 oils. (See pages 153 and 154 for information on how to incorporate omega-3 into your diet.)

Boggy, Swollen Finger

Sometimes a joint becomes enlarged because of swelling of the synovial fluid around it. This can result from an infection that occurred after cutting a cuticle or from rheumatoid arthritis. Initially, the area is soft and boggy. If the inflammation is prolonged, there is an increase in the amount and consistency of the fluid. The fluid thickens and no longer drains efficiently, which increases pressure inside the joint capsule.

This is not a pretty tale. With continued inflammation, powerful enzymes alter the synovial fluid, impairing nutrition and ultimately destroying joint tissues. As the problem progresses, joint surfaces are no longer in their normal alignment, and mechanical injury occurs to the fingers, hand, or wrist. There may be an audible grating or grinding sensation, called *crepitus,* that occurs with motion in this joint or tendon area.

The goal is to try and stay as limber as possible. Simple finger and hand exercises, done several times a day, gently move joints through their full range of motion and keep them strong. The flexing exercises below are great for gentle stretching and strengthening.

FINGER FLEX

Step 1: With your hands in front of you, palms down, spread your fingers and thumbs as far apart as you can, moving one finger at a time.
Step 2: Hold for a count of five and relax.

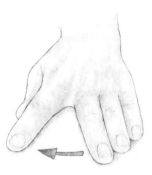

FINGER-JOINT FLEX

Step 1: Gently hold the tip of a finger or thumb with the opposite thumb and index finger and slowly try to bend each single joint by itself, working down the finger toward the palm. Do not force the bending of a joint. Work each finger. Each day repeat this exercise to increase joint flexibility.

Step 2: If any of the joints in your fingers will not straighten completely, do this exercise in reverse. Begin with the finger in the curled position. Uncurl the knuckle joint, then the middle joint, and finally the fingertip. (See more exercise suggestions in the chapter on joints.)

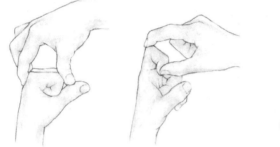

RUBBER–BAND FINGERS

This exercise strengthens the muscles and tendons in your fingers and hand. You'll need rubber bands that are about 1/4 inch wide and 3 inches long.

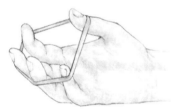

Step 1: Rest your arm on a table palm side up. Place the rubber band around the fingers of one hand at the base of all of your nails.

Step 2: Bend your fingers slightly. Spread the fingers apart; then relax and bring the fingers back together.

NATURAL TREATMENTS FOR ARTHRITIC HANDS

Although osteoarthritis and rheumatoid arthritis are two different ailments, many natural remedies can be useful for both. Any of the following treatments can be used to soothe pain and inflammation associated with arthritis.

Although some herbs are prescribed here, herbal therapy for arthritis is a very large field with many ideas, issues, and theories. These herbs and treatments may help ease the symptoms of arthritis, but they will not be a total solution for the problem. For more information on natural care for arthritis, check in with a practicing specialist.

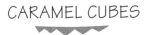

CARAMEL CUBES

This is a wonderful, warming remedy that you can use for spot treatment of pain and inflammation caused by rheumatoid arthritis or osteoarthritis. Red pepper contains aspirin-like ingredients and triggers the body to release pain-relieving chemicals called endorphins. Think of this recipe for finger and thumb joints, wrists, and elbows.

8 ounces (225 g) beeswax
1 cayenne pepper, dried, or 2 fresh cayenne peppers
60 drops (3 ml) St.-John's-wort oil (optional; see recipe on page 158)

Yield: About 16 cubes

(Herbalist Donna Wood Eaton of Cedar Spring Herb Farm in Cape Cod, Massachusetts, shares this recipe with us.)

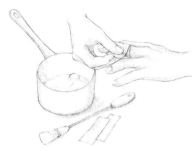

step 2

To make:
1. Melt the beeswax and toss in the cayenne pepper. Simmer slowly for 10 minutes, and then remove the cayenne pepper.
2. Add the St.-John's-wort and stir to blend. Pour mixture, while warm, into empty ice cube trays.
3. Freeze cubes and then transfer them to heavy-duty freezer bags. Label and store in freezer until needed.

To use:
1. Melt 1 cube in a small, old stainless-steel pot.
2. Have toilet tissue and pastry brush at hand. As the beeswax mixture melts, lay the tissue in the palm of your hand and paint the wax onto strips of the tissue. Quickly apply around a finger joint, around a wrist, or on an elbow. To retain the heat, wrap the entire joint in plastic wrap.
3. Allow the beeswax mixture to remain on the area for at least 20 minutes. Repeat at least three times a week to lessen the pain and stiffness of affected joints.

Caution: Fair-skinned folks may find that the skin under the wax turns very red. If this is the case, first coat the area with olive oil or almond oil. If it continues to irritate the skin, discontinue treatment.

PARAFFIN HAND BATH

Paraffin is a waxy substance that holds in heat. This causes the pores to open and allows moisturizers and healing herbs to penetrate the skin. After this treatment, your hands will feel soft, less stiff, and look great.

4 ounces (115 g, or 1 block) paraffin wax
1 ounce (30 ml) olive, almond, or avocado oil
Olive oil (enough to grease a pan)
20 drops (1 ml) essential oil of chamomile, lemon, or geranium (optional)
A few drops of St.-John's-wort oil (see recipe on page 158)or carrot seed oil, enough to coat your hands

To make:

1. Gently heat the paraffin, the olive, almond, or avocado oil, and the essential oil in a double boiler until the paraffin has melted. (Never heat wax directly over an open flame or burner, and never leave wax unattended.)

2. Lightly grease a 10" pie plate or a large glass or ceramic casserole with olive oil (the oil coating will make it easier to clean later). The vessel should be large enough to accommodate your hand.

3. Carefully pour the melted oil and paraffin mixture into the pie plate or casserole. When a thin skin forms on the surface of the wax, the temperature should be right for dipping the hands. Test the wax mixture for temperature comfort with a drop of the wax on the inside of your wrist.

To use:

1. While waiting for the mix to cool, wash your hands and pat dry. Completely coat your fingers and hands with St.-John's-wort oil or carrot seed oil.

2. Dip each hand repeatedly into the melted paraffin mixture, to build up the wax layers. Be sure to include the thumb. The heat and oil will penetrate the muscles and tendons and help relieve stiffness and pain, as well as hydrate the skin.

3. Put each hand into a zip-seal plastic bag. You may need someone to help you if you are doing both hands. Cover both hands with a towel and relax for 15–20 minutes.

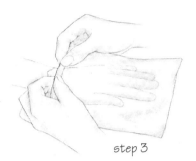

step 3

4. When the time is up, peel away the wax (one hand at a time) by grasping the hand covered with paraffin above wrist and pulling down — the wax should come off in large pieces. (If you've done both hands, you'll need help with this step!) Keep your hand in the plastic bag as you peel away the paraffin to catch all the pieces of wax.

5. Massage and gently stretch your hands.

step 4

PAIN-RELIEVING TEA

In 1835, the buds of the meadowsweet flower were the first discovered source of salicylic acid, the forerunner of aspirin. (If you are sensitive to aspirin, this herb may not be for you.) This tea is a mild sedative and pain reliever and can work wonderfully to relieve the pain of arthritic joints. You can use one or all of these ingredients to create the tea that works for you.

Meadowsweet flower buds
Wintergreen leaves
German chamomile flowers
Lemon or honey (optional)

To make:
Pour boiling water over 1 to 2 teaspoons (5 to 10 ml, or a few pinches) of the dried herbs and steep for 5 to 10 minutes. Strain (or enclose the herbs in a tea ball).

To use:
Flavor with lemon and honey if desired, and drink.

ARTHRITIS RELIEF TEA

Devil's claw, a native of the Kalahari Desert, seems to especially helpful for rheumatic complaints. It has anti-inflammatory and mild analgesic properties with a cortisone-like action for stiff joints. Celery seed helps to counter acid in the blood.

1/2–1 teaspoon (2.5–5 ml) dried rhizome of devil's claw, crushed

1 teaspoon (5 ml) celery seed

1 cup (250 ml) boiling spring water

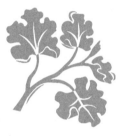

To make:

Boil the herbs in the spring water for 15 minutes. Strain.

To use:

Drink 2 cups a day. Keep it up for a month to judge if it is effective in reducing your arthritis pain.

Variations: Other herbs to try in this tea are crushed valerian root, to relieve swelling and pain and aid sleep; feverfew leaf, to relieve swelling and to help relieve migraine headaches; and blackberry leaf, to relieve joint pain.

Caution: This tea is not suggested during pregnancy or for those with gastric or duodenal ulcers.

MESSÉGUÉ'S VINEGAR RECIPE

This recipe for rose, lavender, or mint vinegar is part of the foot and hand bath regimen recommended by Maurice Mességué for treating osteoarthritis and rheumatoid arthritis (see instructions at right).

Loosely pack 4 to 6 ounces (115 to 170 g) of organically grown red rose petals, lavender flowers, or mint leaves into a quart (liter) jar. Fill jar to top with white vinegar. Cover tightly and steep for 15 days at room temperature in a dark location. Then strain out the petals, seal in a fresh container, and label.

FOOT AND HAND BATHS

A regular regimen, day and night, of foot and hand baths, with particular herbs to treat the pain and impaired mobility of numerous chronic diseases, was the treatment recommended by the popular French herbalist Maurice Mességué. If you would like to try his specific baths for osteoarthritis and rheumatoid arthritis to comfort aching joints and stimulate circulation, be prepared to allow extra time for your hands and feet, twice a day, for at least eight days. Here are the specific guidelines for preparing the baths.

2 quarts (2 liters) water
8 ounces (225 g) crushed or chopped herbs (choose from the lists on page 196)
Rose, lavender, or mint vinegar (see box at left)

Yield: 2 quarts (2 liters)

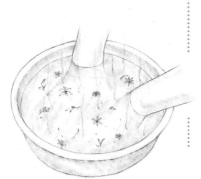

To make:

1. Boil the water for 5 minutes. Cool until just lukewarm.

2. Pour the water into an enamel or plastic container. Drop the crushed or chopped herbs into the water, cover, and allow to steep for 5 hours.

3. Pour the entire mixture into a clean bottle, then cap and refrigerate. This preparation can be stored, rewarmed, and simmered, but not reboiled or diluted. One mixture can be reused for eight days. Refrigerate between uses.

To use:

1. In the morning, before breakfast, heat the infusion as hot as your skin can stand and take a *foot* bath for 8 minutes. In the evening, before supper, reheat the preparation and take a *hand* bath for 8 minutes.

2. After a hand or foot bath, apply rose, lavender, or mint vinegar to stimulate circulation and then a moisturizing cream.

SPECIFIC BATH HERBS
FOR TREATING OSTEOARTHRITIS

Herb	Botanical Latin	Preparation/ Parts Used	Amount
Garlic*	Allium sativum	crushed	1 large, fresh bulb
Nettle	Urtica dioica	leaves and stems, semifresh (if possible), chopped	2 handfuls
Dandelion	Taraxacum officinale	whole plant, semifresh (if possible), chopped	1 handful
Greater celandine	Chelidonium majus	leaves, semifresh (if possible), chopped	1 handful
Meadowsweet	Filipendula ulmaria	flowers, chopped	1 handful
European buttercup	Ranunculus acris	flowers and leaves	1 handful

*Do not use garlic if you have dermatitis.

SPECIFIC BATH HERBS FOR
TREATING RHEUMATOID ARTHRITIS

Herb	Botanical Latin	Preparation/ Parts Used	Amount
Great burdock	Arctium lappa	leaves, chopped	1 handful
Spring heath	Erica spp.	flowers	1 handful
Roman chamomile	Chamaemelum nobile	flowers	12, crushed
Greater celandine	Chelidonium majus	leaves and stems, semifresh (if possible), chopped	1 handful
Couch grass	Agropyron repens	grated roots	1 handful
Common broom	Cytisus scoparius	flowers	1 handful
Lavender	Lavandula spp.	flowers	1 handful
Onion	Allium cepa	grated	1 large

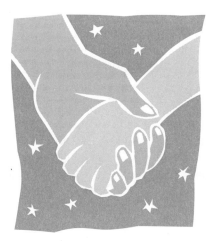

CONCLUSION: Natural Care for the Aging Hand

CONCLUSION

There is no cure for birth and death,
save to enjoy the interval.

— George Santayana

In many ways, our hands mirror and chronicle our life experiences. Abuse your hands, says Henrietta Spencer, and they will give away your most closely guarded secret — your age. Spencer's reasoning is motivation enough to care for the hands that serve us so well and add to our ability to greet, comfort, and express emotion. We need to thank our hands every day for staying with us for a lifetime of service in work and play. I do believe it is never too late to try to make a thing a little bit better. In that spirit, we move forward with information for you on how to maintain and coddle your healthy hands as they mature.

THE AGING HAND

The age of your skin is partially determined by its content of water-soluble collagen. Collagen is a protein necessary for the formation of connective tissue, and it gives skin its flexibility and capacity for absorbing moisture. When the skin becomes thin and less pliable, as it does through the aging process, collagen molecules have oxidized, formed bonds, cross-linked, and become stiffer and less able to swell or absorb moisture. Lines and wrinkles begin to appear. We notice these signs first on the face and neck and on the backs of the hands and arms. Over the years, these areas have been the most vulnerable to the cumulative effect of the sun's rays, which hasten the skin's cellular deterioration.

NATURAL REMEDIES FOR THE AGING HAND

As we grow older and use and abuse our hands, not only does our skin lose its elasticity, but we also become more susceptible to brown spots; bruises and black-and-blue marks; calluses; dry, fragile skin; poor bone health; cold hands; and dilated veins on the backs of the hands. By taking the proper steps to care for our hands now, we can prevent, forestall, or relieve many of these problems.

Skin Elasticity

What it is: As described above, a gradual loss of skin elasticity is one of the hallmarks of the aging hand, and is linked to collagen molecules that have oxidized, formed bonds, cross-linked, and become less able to swell or absorb moisture.

Suggested remedies: New research on collagen and aging skin offers hope that we can delay deterioration in skin elasticity. Studies show that unrefined avocado oil inhibits the activity of the enzyme lysyl oxidase, which is partially responsible for cross-linking collagen. A simple avocado oil, as part of a natural, soluble collagen cream or added to your diet, just may help to slow the clock a bit. Avocado oil also has therapeutic value because it contains the vitamins A, D, and E; is easily absorbed into the skin, as it contains more than 20 percent essential fatty acids; accelerates healing of wounds and eczema; and offers some protection from the sun's damaging ultraviolet rays. It's worth a try.

AVOCADO SKIN CREAM

Oil-Soluble Ingredients

⅓ ounce (9 g) pure unbleached beeswax

¼ cup (60 ml) aromatic, soft green avocado oil

1 teaspoon (5 ml) calendula oil (see recipe on page 129)

1½ teaspoons (7.5 ml) anhydrous lanolin; if there is a lanolin sensitivity, substitute cocoa butter or shea butter

Contents of 1 soy lecithin capsule

Contents of 1 vitamin E capsule

Water-Soluble Ingredients

1 tablespoon (15 ml) distilled water

1 teaspoon (5 ml) glycerin

Pinch of borax

Squeeze of strained lemon juice

10 drops essential oil of geranium, lavender, or patchouli

(Adapted from Margaret Dinsdale's Skin Deep, *Camden House.)*

To make:

1. In a double boiler, gently melt the beeswax.

2. Add the avocado oil, calendula oil, and lanolin (or cocoa butter or shea butter). Stir constantly with a wooden spoon until ingredients are well blended. Remove from heat.

3. In a separate pot, warm the distilled water, glycerin, borax, and lemon juice until all the dry ingredients are dissolved. Remove this mixture from the heat.

4. When the beeswax and oils mixture has cooled, stir in the contents of the lecithin capsule.

5. Slowly add half the water mixture to the beeswax mixture, stirring constantly (or use a hand mixer on a low setting).

6. Stir in the contents of the vitamin E capsule.

7. Slowly add the rest of the water, stirring constantly.

8. Add the essential oil of your choice.

9. When the mixture resembles a mayonnaise texture, stop stirring and pour into a clean glass jar. Do not overdo or the cream will begin to separate. If the cream seems a bit runny, let it cool a minute, stir briefly, and then pour into a glass jar.

10. After it has completely cooled, cap tightly, label, and store in the refrigerator.

To use:

Whenever you notice your hands are looking dry, slightly moisten each hand with water and then rub this cream thoroughly into both.

Brown Spots (or Age Spots)

What they are: Brown spots (sometimes incorrectly called "liver spots"), which usually appear on the backs of the hands, are caused by the cumulative effects of sunlight or chronic bruising of the skin.

Suggested remedies: There are many options among plant remedies that will encourage fading of age spots. Each of us will react differently to the choices, so try a few of these treatments until you find one that works for you.

Sorrel compress. Make a compress from chopped fresh sorrel leaves. Place on a strip of folded gauze and leave on the skin for 15 minutes. Repeat every two or three days.

Chickweed compress. Boil and mash fresh chickweed in soft water and apply as a compress to the hands and arms.

Unrefined avocado oil. This oil contains plant steroids, called sterolins, which have been found to diminish age spots and rebuild collagen. Use the oil in salads and rub into the skin.

Papaya bleach. The natural enzymes in this fruit have been known to bleach brown spots. Mash the fruit and slather over spots. *Caution:* Some sensitive individuals are allergic to papaya. Try a patch test (see page 117) of the mashed fruit first.

Lemon bleach. See recipe for Mrs. Leyel's Lemon-Egg Skin Treatment on page 143.

ONION JUICE AND VINEGAR WASH FOR AGE SPOTS

This is an old folk "cure" for age spots. It can also be used to prevent black-and-blue marks if rubbed on immediately after bruising the skin.

1 teaspoon (5 ml) freshly squeezed onion juice

2 teaspoons (10 ml) organic apple cider vinegar

To make:
Mix onion juice with the vinegar.

To use:
1. Pat this blend on the age spots on the hands at least once a day.
2. Refrigerate leftover mixture.
3. In a few weeks, spots may begin to fade.

TROPICAL BLEACHING LOTION

½ cup (125 ml) distilled water

½ teaspoon (2.5 ml) papaya enzyme powder (see appendix for source)

1 tablespoon (15 ml) xanthan powder

¼ teaspoon (1 ml) Germaben II (available from Cosmetic Supply Company — see "Resources") or 1% vitamin C powder (for short-term storage)

5 drops essential oil of your choice

To make:

1. Pour distilled water into a blender and add the papaya enzyme powder.

2. Turn blender on high and slowly add the xanthan powder and the Germaben II or vitamin C powder. Papaya enzymes smell like cooked beans. To mask this odor, add your favorite essential oil.

To use:

Apply this lotion to the brown spots on your skin. Let dry and then remove with a wet sponge or cloth, and rinse thoroughly. After the treatment, your skin will feel soft and moist. Follow up with a moisturizer.

Yield: Makes 4 ounces (115 g)

(Shared by Nikolaus J. Smeh, Natural Skincare Institute.)

Bruising Easily

What it is: Almost everyone who has *TMB* ("too many birthdays," a term employed by Dr. Joseph Bark, a dermatologist) will, at some time or another as he or she grows older, suffer from black-and-blue marks on the backs of hands or arms. These superficial bruises are caused when the collagen support network under the skin has begun to weaken and the skin becomes fragile. Some people describe this skin as "tissue-paper-skin." Prolonged use of steroid medications may be a factor here. Because of a decrease in skin density, tiny vessels in the outer skin are now more susceptible to physical impact and damage by sunlight.

Suggested remedies: Take extra care in using heat, cold, massage, and adhesives on fragile skin. They can easily cause damage to blood vessels in delicate skin and result in bruising.

Avoid aspirin if you bruise easily. Aspirin thins the blood and may encourage bleeding under the skin. Also try to avoid adhesive tape bandages on the hands and arms. If you need to bandage a wound, wrap the area with a gauze-type dressing.

First aid. At first impact that may result in a superficial bruise, apply firm pressure to the injured spot and maintain this pressure for at least 5 minutes. This procedure will allow the blood to clot in place.

Onion and vinegar wash. Immediately after an impact that may cause a superficial bruise, apply an onion juice and vinegar wash (see recipe at left).

Arnica/witch hazel compress. Make a compress using 1 part arnica tincture (see recipe below) to 10 parts non-distilled witch hazel extract to relieve pain and treat the bruise.

ARNICA TINCTURE

Arnica has pain-relieving and anti-inflammatory properties and is a very helpful herb for black-and-blue marks and bruises.

2 ounces (60 g) arnica flowers, dried and crushed

2 cups (500 ml) 70- to 100-proof grain alcohol

To make:
1. Put the crushed flowers in a jar.
2. Cover with alcohol. Seal.
3. Shake daily for seven days.
4. Strain off flowers.

To use:
Use as a first-aid remedy for bruises, sprains, and aching joints. Dab directly on skin of affected area with a bit of cotton.

Caution: Do not apply arnica directly on broken skin.

A TALE OF ARNICA:
DON'T LEAVE HOME WITHOUT IT!

The setting: Picture yourself at the start of a vacation. You are on a jet plane that is taking you to a sunny destination. It's not a direct flight because you wanted to be economical. Now, because of fog, the first landing is delayed and the touchdown is a bit bumpy. Connecting passengers are in a hurry. The gentleman across the aisle in front of you jumps up and throws open the overhead compartment. Sailing out is a hard-bodied briefcase (the kind that can crush a Timex watch!).

This durable piece of luggage lands squarely on the back of your preferred hand, prompting the development of a new mountain on your anatomy and the beginnings of an artist's palette against the normally soft hues of your skin.

The reaction: A loud ouch! Later, a bag of ice cubes provided by the steward brings some relief. However, a boarding passenger arrives to take the seat next to you. He notices that you are reading a book on medicinal herbs and volunteers that he never travels without his plant remedies. He has arnica extract in his bag and proceeds to dab it lightly on your bruised hand. Within 5 minutes, the newly formed mountain is returning to normal. Before the second landing, he reapplies more arnica and the black-and-blue appearance begins to disappear. At final touchdown, the steward returns to ask about the injured hand and cannot believe that there is no bruise. (But, the spot was still tender!)

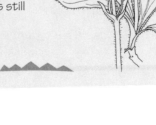

COMFREY COMPRESS

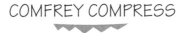

Comfrey has been used for centuries to treat skin problems. One of this plant's major ingredients is allantoin, which promotes skin repair. An old-time remedy for bruises is a comfrey compress.

3 tablespoons (45 ml) dried comfrey root or powder, crushed
2 cups (500 ml) boiling water

To make:
Add the comfrey root or powder to the boiling water and simmer gently for 10 minutes.

To use:
1. Soak a bit of gauze or other suitable material in this solution and place it on the bruise.
2. If done quickly after the impact, skin discoloration may be prevented.
3. Repeat two or three times during the day.
Caution: Drinking comfrey tea is not recommended, as it has other ingredients that may be toxic to the liver.

Callused Hands

What it is: As we age, we have less cushioning tissue than normal and are thus more susceptible to calluses. One particular type of callus is often found on the palms of people who use assistive walking devices such as canes or walkers. The roughening and thickening is caused by the constant pressure and friction on the palm. Blisters may precede calluses. This change in the outside surface of the skin can cause tenderness in the tissues beneath.
Suggested remedy: Try the "Green Rub" recipe on page 206 as a mild abrasive wash to gently smooth calluses on the palms.

GREEN RUB

1–2 tablespoons (15–30 ml) cornmeal
1 tablespoon (15 ml) fresh mashed avocado or avocado oil

To make:
Mix both ingredients in a small bowl till they form a meal-like mixture.
To use:
1. Place the mixture in the palm of your hand. Rub both hands together and work the gritty and emollient meal into the calluses and up and around the fingers.
2. Repeat once or twice a week.

Cold Hands

What they are: Cold hands are often caused by circulatory problems, although coronary artery disease, illness, and sedentary lifestyles are other causes frequently seen in older populations. One unusual cause of cold hands is called Raynaud's phenomenon, which causes spasms of the small arteries and veins in the hands and the feet. Raynaud's is an exaggerated constrictive response to cold resulting in cold, white, numb fingers, ears, and toes, which may later swell and turn blue.

Suggested remedies: There are several simple ways to enhance circulation to your extremities. Maintain a high core body temperature and keep your torso warm. Use insulated gloves and shoes or boots for cold-weather activities. Treat yourself to regular massages and avoid smoking.

Vitamin and mineral supplements. Supplement your diet with calcium, a vasodilator. You can also try increasing the amount of vitamin C in your diet. Research has shown that vitamin C may help our internal body thermostats adjust more easily to temperature changes.

Ginkgo supplements. The leaves of this ancient tree have properties that act as circulatory stimulants, improving blood flow to the hands, feet, and brain. Ask your healthcare provider about the use of this compound. Capsules are available in 40 to 60 mg sizes. The suggested dosage is to begin with 1 capsule and work up to 120 mg a day. (You can also infuse ginkgo biloba and drink as an herbal tea.)

Hawthorn extract. Hawthorn flowers and berries improve circulation in coronary arteries and increase blood flow without raising blood pressure. This herb may help those with cold hands because it dilates blood vessels and improves capillary strength. Take a capsule supplement containing a 2 percent standardized extract of hawthorn berry, 100 to 250 mg, twice a day (but check in with your healthcare provider first). You can also try Hawthorn Flower Tea (see recipe on page 208).

CONDITIONING FOR COLD-WEATHER ACTIVITIES

This is a simple conditioning treatment developed by Dr. Murray Hamlet, director of the Cold Research Division, U.S. Army Institute of Environmental Medicine, Natick, Massachusetts. It offers poor-circulation sufferers possibilities for cold-weather activities without pain.

This procedure is time consuming, but it involves only easy steps to natural conditioning. The treatment helps to reverse the body's constrictor message to peripheral vessels, even under cold-weather conditions. Results can last a "number of years" and relapses can be reversed by repeating the procedure.

Step 1: Find two containers large enough for both hands to be immersed. Fill one with 104°F (40°C) water and the other with 108°F (42°C) water. Place the 108°F (42°C) water in a cold area such as a cold room, basement, or outdoors; place the 104°F (40°C) in a warm room.

Step 2: Dress lightly as you would indoors. In the warm room, immerse both hands in the 104°F (40°C) water for 2 to 5 minutes.

Step 3: Wrap your hands in a towel. Go to the cold area and immerse both hands in the container of 108°F (42°C) water for 10 minutes.

Step 4: Return indoors and place hands again in the basin of 104°F (40°C) water for 2 to 5 minutes. (A helper will have to keep the water at the correct temperature for you.)

Step 5: This is the tough part — repeat this procedure three to six times a day for about 50 days.

HAWTHORN FLOWER TEA

1–2 teaspoons (5–10 ml) hawthorn, flowers and leaves
1 cup (250 ml) boiling water

To make:
Pour boiling water over the flowers and leaves and steep for 5 to 10 minutes in a covered cup.

To use:
Dose is 1 cup.

Dilated Veins

What it is: As the skin ages and loses part of its collagen support and oil-producing system, it begins to look thinner and more fragile. Sometimes the veins in the extremities grow less efficient in pumping blood back to the heart. The blood begins to pool, dilates the veins on the back of the hand, and can leak into the skin, depositing a purplish pigment.

Suggested remedies: Several herbal treatments can be used to both discourage and heal dilated veins. To keep the skin supple and less prone to the purplish pigment deposits caused by dilated veins, use avocado oil or the Avocado Skin Cream recipe (page 200) regularly.

SPRING DANDELION COMPRESS

Use this to soothe dilated veins on hands.

Young shoots of dandelion leaves, finely chopped (collect shoots before the plant flowers)
Boiling water
Calendula oil (see recipe on page 129)

To make:
Simmer the finely chopped leaves for 5 minutes and allow to cool until the liquid is lukewarm.

To use:
1. Dip a clean cloth into this infusion. Squeeze out the excess liquid and wrap your hands with this compress.
2. Cover with a towel. Relax for 10 minutes.
3. Afterward, apply a thin coat of calendula oil to your hands.

COLTSFOOT, CHAMOMILE, AND YARROW COMPRESS

Coltsfoot is known as a demulcent and soothing herb; chamomile flowers are noted for their anti-inflammatory and wound-healing properties; and yarrow is known to tone veins and prevent blood clots. Choose one or a blend of all of these ingredients, and make a large batch ahead of time to keep on-hand.

1 teaspoon (5 ml) colts-
   foot leaves, German
   chamomile flowers,
   and/or yarrow flower
   and leaf, chopped
1 cup (250 ml) boiling
   water
Almond or avocado oil
   (optional)

To make:

1. Pour the boiling water over the herbs and allow to steep for 20 minutes. Strain the herbs, reserving the herb liquid.

2. When the infusion has cooled to lukewarm, pour into a small bowl.

3. You can double or triple this recipe and make enough for a week by storing the extra liquid in a covered container in the refrigerator. Warm gently as needed.

To use:

1. Rinse your hands in warm water and pat dry. If your hands are very dry, coat them with a thin layer of almond or avocado oil before applying the compress.

2. Dip a tea towel in the liquid and wring it a bit so that it does not drip. Wrap both hands. Cover with a second towel. Relax. Listen to pleasant music for 10 to 15 minutes.

3. Don't rinse away the infused liquid afterward. If desired, apply a moisturizer to your hands. Don't use any hand lotions that contain alcohol.

Dry Skin

What it is: The body's natural production of oil slows over the years. As our hormonal levels change — for women, as estrogen decreases — rough, dry skin develops because there is little hormonal stimulation to the sebaceous glands, which shrink in size and produce less oil. There is less of an oily surface, then, to attract moisture from the surrounding environment. Sun, wind, low humidity, artificial heating, air conditioning, air travel, and harsh detergent or antibacterial soaps further dehydrate and injure the skin. As we age, dry skin is most often noticeable on the backs of our hands and on our elbows.

Did you know that dryness does not cause wrinkles? Instead, dryness can accentuate creases and furrows. Dermatologists are in almost total agreement that it is exposure to the sun that damages the supporting elastic and collagen fibers in the dermis. To protect yourself and your hands from the sun, use hand creams, sunscreen, long sleeves, and gloves.

Suggested remedies: To increase skin moisture and soothe dry skin, protect yourself from skin-drying agents and use moisturizers frequently. Following are some home tips for improving humidity and moisture in skin and hands:

- Leave toilet seats up. (Don't laugh!)
- Store about 1 inch (2.5 cm) of water in the bathtub.
- Let aquarium fish be your pets.
- Buy a cool-mist humidifier for the bedroom.
- Wash with a mild, unscented, superfatted soap. Harsh soaps strip away natural oils and perfumed soaps contain alcohol, which is drying. Use lukewarm water and be brief. Hot water depletes moisture from the hands.
- Blot hands dry. Vigorous rubbing creates tiny tears in fragile skin. Keep a bottle of moisturizer near the sink and use it often. Apply a moisturizer each time your hands are in water. Spread the cream over slightly moist skin. Have small containers of moisturizer to carry with you away from home.
- Protect hands with the appropriate gloves when doing wet work.
- Drink plenty of bottled water and fresh fruit juice.
- Before going outdoors, apply at least an SPF 15 sunscreen to your hands.

HONEY OINTMENT

This easy-to-make ointment will heal and rehydrate hands and arms. Honey is antibacterial and retains moisture. It's also wonderful to smooth on nicks, bruises, and minor burns to encourage healing.

1 ounce (30 g) beeswax
1 cup (250 ml) olive, almond, or apricot oil
1/3 cup (75 ml) honey
Up to 60 drops (3 ml) essential oils of rose geranium, lavender, or bergamot (optional)

Yield: Makes about six 2-ounce (60 ml) jars

(This recipe is shared by beekeepers Stephen and Deb Pouech of Herbs 'n Honey in Stafford Springs, Connecticut.)

To make:

1. In a double boiler, melt the beeswax. Stir periodically to facilitate melting. This process should take approximately 10 minutes.

2. Add the oil to the melted beeswax. Stir until thoroughly blended.

3. Remove from heat and let cool slightly. Add honey and stir until incorporated. If desired, add essential oils now.

4. Pour into jars. Wait until room temperature to cap. Label and date. Jars can be stored at room temperature.

To use:

Smooth on affected areas.

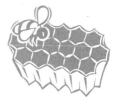

LOTIONS VERSUS MOISTURIZERS

The purpose of lotions, creams, and moisturizers is to increase the water content in skin. The simple difference among them is that creams and lotions work by increasing the ability of the skin to retain water. Moisturizers seal in moisture.

SHEA BUTTER HAND AND
ELBOW CREAM AND SUNSCREEN

¾ cup (180 ml) hot water (150°F, or 66°C)

1 teaspoon (5 ml) lemon juice

½ teaspoon (2.5 ml) xanthan powder

1 teaspoon (5 ml) phospholipids (available from many cosmetic companies, including Cosmetic Supply Company — see "Resources")

3 teaspoons (15 ml) hot shea butter or avocado oil (150°F, or 66°C)

½ teaspoon (50 drops) essential oils or vitamins of your choice (optional)

Titanium dioxide (optional; this compound is available from Cosmetic Supply Company — see "Resources")

(Shared by Nikolaus J. Smeh, Natural Skincare Institute.)

To make:

1. Mix the hot water, lemon juice, and xanthan powder in a kitchen blender.

2. Add the phospholipids and the hot shea butter or avocado oil to the mixture in the blender and blend again for 1 minute.

3. Stir in the essential oils or vitamins if desired.

4. Let cool to room temperature, then blend again for 30 seconds.

5. If adding titanium dioxide (see below), add now and blend briefly.

6. Put into small glass or plastic jars and let stand overnight. In the morning, you will have an easy, spreadable, state-of-the-art liposome cream.

7. If you do not add preservatives, you will need to store this cream in the refrigerator.

To use:

Smooth onto skin before venturing out into the sun. An outdoor person involved in golf, tennis, gardening, or walking will benefit from a twice-daily application of this moisturizing sunscreen, a sun hat, long sleeves, and gloves.

For sun protection: Shea butter itself has an SPF of 4. However, for greater protection, consider adding titanium dioxide (a natural mineral). For an SPF of 15, add 1½ tablespoons (23 ml) of titanium dioxide. For every 1% of SPF that you want to increase, add ½ teaspoon (2.5 ml) more.

Osteoporosis

What it is: Almost twenty million people have some form of osteoporosis. Bone mass stops developing at age thirty-five and bones slowly start losing the calcium that has been stored in the skeleton. When the reserves are depleted and not restocked, the bones of our frame become porous and brittle. In a fall, the bones of our wrists and forearms become more susceptible to fracture or breaking as a result of poor bone health.

Suggested remedies: Stop smoking! Women who smoke have lower estrogen levels and undergo menopause at an earlier age. Early menopause sets up more years without the bone-strengthening protection of natural estrogen, which slows the depletion of calcium from bone.

There are a number of other simple ways you can protect yourself from calcium depletion and osteoporosis:

- If you are taking calcium supplements, take them with yogurt or milk and spread out the dosage during the day and before bed (see page 41 for information on dosage).
- Eat foods that are high in acids: citrus fruits, tomatoes, cranberry juice, and vinegars. These foods improve calcium absorption.
- Cut down on salt or sodium. At the same time sodium is excreted in the urine, so is calcium.
- Avoid carbonated soda beverages (including diet sodas). These contain high levels of phosphates and interfere with calcium absorption.
- Drink six 8-ounce glasses of water a day. Water helps to carry nutrients, hormones, and oxygen throughout the body and flushes out waste products. As we age, we seem to lose our sense of thirst. If we don't replenish fluids lost through normal excretion, the body is forced to pull essential water from the liver and kidneys. This can lead to other problems.
- Keep caffeine consumption down to no more than 16 ounces a day. Excess caffeine depletes the body's vitamin C, calcium, zinc, potassium, and B vitamins.
- Schedule a program of regular weight-bearing exercise. Walking every day is the single most important thing

you can do for whole-body health. According to Maggie Lettvin — teacher, writer, TV personality, and expert on the body as a machine — the reason osteoporosis can result in broken wrists and arms is that we have not kept our hips and leg bones strong: "For want of a nail, the shoe was lost. Everything leads to something else." If you are able, include working with light weights to maintain the strength in your hands, wrists, and arms. It is only through movement that the synovial fluid brings nourishment to the joint cartilage and that waste products are eliminated.

◆ Be aware of medications that reduce bone density: aluminum-containing antacids, steroids such as pred- nisone and cortisone, diuretics, anticoagulants, and anticonvulsants.

Bone stock. Using bone stock as a base for soups and other dishes is an easy and inexpensive way to add calcium to your diet, and it's much tastier than elephant-size calcium pills. See the recipe to the right. Below are some general hints for finding, storing, and preparing bones:

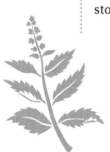

◆ Keep a plastic bag in the freezer and collect various bones for your soups. One broth can be from leftover chicken or turkey carcasses, another from beef bones, and another from the bones of fish.

◆ Put chicken and turkey bones into the cooking water as is. Other larger bones need to be split. Ask your grocer to do this for you.

◆ Inquire at your fish market for free bones left after fil- leting. Ask for skeletons from the seafood they think will make a good fish stock. After cooking, you can put these through a blender and make a super chowder by adding milk to the recipe.

MAGGIE LETTVIN'S SOUP BONE STOCK

This recipe for bone stock gives you a simple way to add calcium to your diet and improve your bone health. It can be used to flavor not only soup but also rice, vegetables, and a variety of other dishes.

2 pounds (32 ounces) bones

2 quarts (2 liters) distilled water or spring water (or enough to cover bones)

1 cup (250 ml) tomatoes or ¼ cup (60 ml) apple cider vinegar

1 medium onion, halved

½ band dried kelp seaweed (optional)

(Adapted from Maggie Lettvin's Food Strategy Book.*)*

To make:

1. Combine all ingredients in a large stainless stockpot. Cover and bring to a boil. If you use the apple cider vinegar, you will notice a vinegary smell. Cook until the smell disappears. This acid is leaching the calcium from the bones into the soup.

2. Lower the heat and simmer covered 2 to 3 hours. Do not cook too briskly.

3. Strain the stock to remove all bits of bone. Chill.

4. As the fat solidifies on the top of the soup stock, skim it off with a spoon.

To use:

The broth is now ready for you to add more vegetables and seasonings as a base for your other creations. I like to pour some of the strained, seasoned broth into ice cube trays to keep in the freezer for flavoring rice and other dishes.

APPENDIX A:
A Guide to Natural
and Herbal Ingredients

A NOTE ABOUT BOTANICAL NAMES

Before we delve into natural treatments or remedies for preserving and healing our hands, it is well to understand a bit about nature's pharmacy. Throughout the book, I have used the common names of the plants in the recipes. The problem with common names is that one plant may have many common names, or that several plants may have the same name. (For example, greater celandine and wartweed are the same flower, and *Chamaemelum nobile* and *Matricaria recutita* are both called chamomile.)

The botanical or scientific name of a plant, however, is recognized internationally, in all languages, and should refer to just one particular plant. This botanical name usually consists of two Latin words. The first designates the genus (a group of plants with a distinctive set of similar characteristics) to which the plant belongs. The second word denotes the plant's species (a smaller, even more similar group within the genus). The species name often refers to the place of origin or one outstanding characteristic of the plants in that group. For example, the botanical Latin name for black currant is *Ribes nigrum*. *Ribes* indicates that it belongs to the genus *Ribes*, and *nigrum*, its species name, means "black."

In a remedy, it is important to use the specific medicinal plant that is called for. It has properties that have been proven either through traditional folk usage or research studies. Other species within the same plant family may not have the same active principles necessary to effect healing. If all of the species within a genus are appropriate, rather than one particular species, the abbreviation "spp." (meaning "species") will follow the genus name, meaning that you can choose any species within that genus to use in preparing the remedy.

This glossary briefly describes the natural and herbal ingredients called for in the recipes. You can find these ingredients in herb shops, garden centers, natural-food stores, or via mail-order suppliers. And, if you are out in the woods, fields, or herb gardens studying these plants, be sure to take along a few regional field guides to help you identify them.

ACACIA SHRUB OR TREE (*Acacia senegal*)
Also Known As: Gum-arabic tree
Parts Used: Gummy substance secreted from the bark
Properties: Gum acacia is soluble in water, forming a mucilage-type paste; because its contents include calcium, magnesium, and potassium, the gum can be used with other herbs as a nutritious emulsifier and a soothing demulcent to cover or wrap inflamed tissues.

ALKANET (*Anchusa officinalis* or *Alkanna tinctoria*)
Also Known As: Anchusa, Dyer's bugloss
Parts Used: Rind of the root soaked in oil or alcohol
Properties: Colorant or dye, astringent

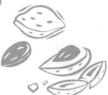

ALMOND, SWEET (*Prunus dulcis* var. *dulcis*)
Parts Used: Nut or seed, powder, oil pressed from the seed.
Properties: Demulcent, emollient, nutritive (a source of iron, calcium, potassium, copper, zinc, vitamin E, biotin, plus 18 of the 20 amino acids needed for healthy growth), skin softener; often used in body oils and lotions.

ALOE (*Aloe vera*)
Parts Used: Gel from the succulent leaves; some suppliers also sell aloe vera "juice," which does *not* have the same healing properties as the gel.
Properties: Demulcent, antibacterial, antibiotic; source of allantoin; useful for healing cuts and wounds, as an analgesic for mild pain, and for soothing sunburn.
Caution: Not recommended for use during pregnancy.

ANGELICA *(Angelica archangelica)*

Parts Used: Leaves, stems and stalks, seeds, or dried root

Properties: Aromatic, flavoring (anglica is one of the herbs used to flavor vermouth), diaphoretic, carminative, circulatory stimulant

Caution: Not recommended for use during pregnancy or by diabetics.

APPLE CIDER VINEGAR

Properties: Rich in potassium and trace minerals; used as a preservative, antibacterial, antiseptic, cleanser, and menstruum for herbal medicine; has a slightly acid pH similar to skin.

APRICOT OIL

Properties: A light, fine oil useful for sensitive or delicate skin; helpful in healing damaged skin cells; skin softener; rich in vitamins A and B; may be used as a substitute for sweet almond oil.

ARNICA *(Arnica montana)*

Also Known As: Leopard's bane

Parts Used: Flowers, root

Properties: Reduces inflammation and external signs of bruising; applied to sprains, aches, and pains.

Caution: Not recommended for use on broken or lacerated skin. Redheads and blondes may develop sun sensitivity as a result of exposure to arnica, although this is a rare occurrence.

ASTRAGALUS *(Astragalus membranaceus)*

Also Known As: In Chinese, *Huang-qi*

Parts Used: Dried root

Properties: Boosts immune system health; antiviral, antibacterial, diuretic.

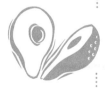

AVOCADO *(Persea americana)*

Parts Used: Seed, oil from the pulp of the pear

Properties: Skin-friendly moisturizer; rebuilds skin collagen; diminishes age spots; contains vitamins A, D, and E; useful for soothing sunburn.

BAKING SODA (Sodium bicarbonate)
Parts Used: Powder
Properties: Alkaline skin conditioner; soothes minor skin irritations, including bee stings and itching.

BASIL, SWEET (*Ocimum basilicum*)
Parts Used: Leaves and stems
Properties: Contains vitamins A and C; fly deterrent; aromatic, carminative, antispasmodic; fresh juice can be used on bee stings.

BEARBERRY (*Arctostaphylos uva-ursi*)
Also Known As: Uva-ursi
Parts Used: Leaves
Properties: Astringent and diuretic when used in a tea infusion; useful for inflammatory diseases of the urinary tract, fluid retention, and backache.
Caution: Not recommended for use during pregnancy or for those with kidney disorders.

BEESWAX
Properties: Obtained from the honeycomb of honeybees; holds fatty oils in emulsion in moisturizing creams and lotions; natural beeswax is dark yellow.

BENZOIN (*Styrax benzoin*)
Also Known As: Gum benzoin
Parts Used: Tree resin, tincture of benzoin
Properties: Antiseptic and astringent; used to heal inflamed, irritated, and cracked skin bothered by the environment; improves skin elasticity; cosmetic fixative and preservative of fats.

BERGAMOT (*Monarda didyma*)
Also Known As: Bee balm, Oswego tea
Parts Used: Young leaves for tea, essential oil
Properties: Antiseptic and carminative; has a strong citrus fragrance; nice in a carrier oil blend with lavender and patchouli.
Caution: Direct sunlight can cause darkening of skin to which bergamot has been applied.

BLACKBERRY *(Rubus allegheniensis)*
Parts Used: Leaves, berries, root, bark
Properties: Powerful astringent and tonic; useful as a tea or wash for wounds.

BLEACH (Sodium hypochlorite 5.25% and inert ingredients)
Properties: A strong oxidizer, disinfectant, stain remover, deodorizer.
Caution: Dilute before using.

BORAGE *(Borago officinalis)*
Parts Used: Leaves and flowering tops
Properties: Demulcent, mucilage, and emollient. Borage oil contains two important fatty acids, gamma-linolenic acid (GLA) and linoleic acid, that encourage healthy hair, nails, and skin.

BORAX (Sodium borate)
Parts Used: White, crystalline, mineral powder
Properties: Antiseptic, emulsifier, and buffering agent for moisturizers, scrubs, bath salts.

BROOM, COMMON *(Cytisus scoparius)*
Parts Used: Tops of the flowering branches
Properties: Brush-like branches can be diuretic in infusions, tinctures, or decoctions.
Caution: Not recommended for use during pregnancy, by nursing mothers, or by those with high blood pressure.

BURDOCK *(Arctium lappa)*
Parts Used: Crushed seeds (fruits) inside sticky burs, root, leaves
Properties: Adaptogen, demulcent, diaphoretic, diuretic, bitter; cleanses body system to relieve skin problems; useful as an aid in treatment of arthritis; contains B-vitamins, iron, and sulfur.
Caution: Not recommended for use during pregnancy or by nursing mothers.

BUTTERCUP *(Ranunculus acris)*

Also Known As: Upright meadow crowfoot

Parts Used: Whole herb, flowers, and leaves

Properties: Caustic; juice can be used to remove warts.

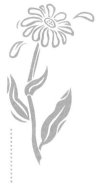

BUTTERMILK

See Milk.

CALENDULA *(Calendula officinalis)*

Also Known As: Pot marigold

Parts Used: Flower heads, leaves

Properties: Can be prepared as a tea, tincture, cream, or poultice for healing wounds, stings, inflamed skin around fingernails, chapped skin, and windburn.

CARROT *(Daucus carota* var. *sativa)*

Parts Used: Whole herb, mashed; seeds and root; seed oil

Properties: Rich in beta carotene and antioxidant vitamins and minerals; diuretic, carminative, stimulant; a 10 percent dilution of the seed oil can be used to prevent scar formation and improve skin texture.

CASTOR OIL

Properties: A heavy, protective, soothing oil; laxative; helps to seal in moisture in skin preparations.

CAYENNE PEPPER *(Capsicum annuum)*

Also Known As: Chile pepper

Parts Used: Fruit, ripe and dried

Properties: Contains capsaicin, a powerful local stimulant and rubefacient that increases the flow of blood and oxygenation of body cells, produces natural warmth, and functions as an antiseptic; can be prepared as a tincture to treat cold hands and feet.

CEDAR, RED *(Thuja plicata)*

Parts Used: Fan-like braches of young trees

Properties: Antifungal and antibacterial; stimulates immune response; leaves are often used for incense; can be prepared as a tincture to treat nail fungus.

CEDAR, WHITE (*Thuja occidentalis*)

Also Known As: Arborvitae

Parts Used: New growth, leafy, terminal twigs

Properties: Antibacterial, antiviral, diuretic, nervine; can be used to treat warts, skin fungus, and itchy skin disorders.

Caution: Not recommended for use during pregnancy or by nursing mothers.

CELANDINE, GREATER (*Chelidonium majus*)

Also Known As: Wartweed

Parts Used: Juice obtained from plants

Properties: Bitter, antifungal, and antispasmodic; the orange-colored acrid juice of the fresh plants can be dripped on warts and corns.

CELERY (*Apium graveolens* var. *dulce*)

Parts Used: Whole herb, seed, juice, liquid extract

Properties: Contains iron, potassium, sodium, and phosphorus; diuretic, carminative, urinary antiseptic, and anti-inflammatory; can help ease stiffness and muscular pain.

CHAMOMILE (*Chamaemelum nobile, Matricaria recutita*)

Parts Used: Flower heads, essential oil

Properties: German chamomile *(M. recutita)* and Roman chamomile *(C. nobile)*, the two types of chamomile most often used medicinally, have almost identical properties (although you should use the one called for in a recipe if specified). Anti-inflammatory, antimicrobial, antiseptic, analgesic, mild tranquilizer, and bitter; can be prepared as a tea, a compress, and an infused oil.

CHICKWEED (*Stellaria media*)

Parts Used: Whole herb

Properties: A demulcent, emollient, vulnerary, and anti-itch herb; cools, soothes, and relieves skin irritation.

CITRUS SEED EXTRACT

Properties: Bitter, antiseptic, and calming extract; try using one to two drops in skin cream.

CLOVER, RED *(Trifolium pratense)*

Parts Used: Flower heads

Properties: Alterative and anti-inflammatory; useful for eczema, skin diseases, and sores that refuse to heal; promotes healthy healing of tissue.

COCOA BUTTER

Properties: The fat is used in making ointments and cosmetic creams; has a chocolate aroma.

COCONUT BUTTER AND OIL

Properties: Coconut oil comes from the coconut palm *(Cocos nucifera)*. *Copra*, coconut meat, is called coconut butter. Coconut oil and butter are skin softeners; often used in emollient ointments and creams.

COD-LIVER OIL

Properties: A valuable source of vitamins A and D; also used to heal burns and wounds.

COLTSFOOT *(Tussilago farfara)*

Also Known As: Coughwort

Parts Used: Whole herb, leaves, flowers, root

Properties: Demulcent, bitter, anti-inflammatory, and expectorant.

Caution: Not recommended for use during pregnancy or by nursing mothers.

COMFREY *(Symphytum officinale)*

Also Known As: Knitbone

Parts Used: Leaves, root

Properties: Demulcent and mildly astringent; source of allantoin, which helps emollient action; leaves are used as external remedies for sprains, swelling, and bruises and as a poultice or a salve ingredient for cuts, boils, and abscesses; useful for any external area of inflammatory swelling.

CORN *(Zea mays)*

Parts Used: Cornmeal, cornstarch, corn oil, corn silk

Properties: Cornmeal can be used as a mild abrasive; cornstarch can be used as a thickener; corn oil can be used as an emollient for nails and skin; corn silk, the pistils of the flowers, can be used as a diuretic when taken as a tea.

COUCH-GRASS *(Agropyron repens)*

Also Known As: Twitch grass

Parts Used: Rhizome or underground stem

Properties: Diuretic and demulcent; recommended for gout and rheumatism.

CREAM

See Milk.

CURRANT, BLACK *(Ribes nigrum)*

Parts Used: Fruit, leaves, bark, root

Properties: Astringent, diuretic, anti-inflammatory, and diaphoretic.

DANDELION *(Taraxacum officinale)*

Parts Used: Dried root, leaves, stem

Properties: Contains vitamins A, B, and C, and minerals; diuretic; soothing to insect bites; can be used to treat warts or as a coffee substitute.

DEVIL'S CLAW *(Harpagophytum procumbens)*

Parts Used: Rhizome or underground stem

Properties: Mild analgesic and anti-inflammatory; cortisone-like action for stiff arthritic joints or itchy skin conditions.

Caution: Not recommended for use during pregnancy or by those with gastric or duodenal ulcers.

DOCK, YELLOW *(Rumex crispus)*

Also Known As: Curled dock

Parts Used: Leaves, root

Properties: Astringent; leaves are rich in vitamins A and C; used as an alterative tonic for eruptions of chronically dry and itchy skin, boils, and shingles; remedy for stinging nettle rash.

ECHINACEA *(Echinacea angustifolia, E. purpurea)*
Also Known As: Coneflower
Parts Used: Rhizome and the whole plant
Properties: Antiseptic, anti-inflammatory, antimicrobial, vulnerary, tonic; stimulates immune response; raises the white blood cell count and increases the body's resistance to disease; useful for any skin disorder.

ELDER, BLACK *(Sambucus nigra)*
Parts Used: Bark, leaves, flowers, berries
Properties: An infusion of the fresh leaves works as a mosquito repellent; bruised leaves worn in a sun hat will keep away flies; the berries contain vitamin C and iron and are an old cure, in a cordial, for the common cold; elder-flower water is used to clear the skin of freckles; the hot tea is a remedy for colds, sore throat, and the flu; and the cold tea is a remedy for chapped hands.

EVENING PRIMROSE *(Oenothera biennis)*
Parts Used: Bark of flower stems, leaves, seeds, seed oil
Properties: Oil contains gamma linolenic acid; oil can be applied externally with vitamin E to protect the moisture balance of the skin and help in treating eczema or soft or brittle fingernails. The leaves and flowers, in a poultice, aid abscesses and boils.
Caution: Not recommended for use by those with epilepsy.

FALSE SOLOMON'S SEAL *(Smilacina racemosa)*
Parts Used: Crushed, fresh, or powdered root
Properties: Astringent and demulcent; an excellent poultice for bruises and inflammations.

FEVERFEW *(Tanacetum parthenium)*
Parts Used: Fresh leaf, powder
Properties: Anti-inflammatory, fever reducer, bitter, carminative; capsulated, dried leaf is a treatment for migraine headaches; crushed leaves can be applied to aching muscles and joints. New research suggests the possibility that feverfew may offer relief for those suffering from osteoarthritis and inflammatory rheumatism.
Caution: Not recommended for use during pregnancy or by those taking contraceptive pills.

FLAX *(Linum usitatissimum)*

Also Known As: Linseed

Parts Used: Seeds, oil from seeds

Properties: Emollient, demulcent; richer in omega-3 oils than fish; crushed seeds offer healing mucilage for poultices to treat abscesses and boils by reducing irritation, pain, and inflammation.

GARLIC *(Allium sativum)*

Parts Used: Bulb, fresh cloves, juice

Properties: Antiseptic, antibiotic, anti-viral, antiallergy, anticoagulant, detoxifier, carminative, diaphoretic, and stimulant; may protect the heart and nervous system, enhance the body's immune system, decrease the side effects of drug therapies for cancer, and more. The therapeutically active ingredient in garlic is the smelly *allicin*. Garlic also contains amino acids, selenium, sulfur, B-vitamins, and minerals.

Caution: Fresh garlic juice on the skin can cause blistering.

GERANIUM *(Pelargonium* spp.)

Parts Used: Leaves, essential oil

Properties: Essential oil of geranium is refreshing, fragrant, relaxing, and can act as an antidepressant; its actions are mildly astringent, antibacterial, and antifungal; balances moisture in dry or mature skin; softens wrinkles by promoting new cell generation.

Caution: Do not use where skin is exposed to strong sunlight or during early pregnancy.

GINGER *(Zingiber officinale)*

Parts Used: Dried rhizome, oil, powder

Properties: Anti-inflammatory, circulatory stimulant, and antiseptic; controls nausea; drinking ginger tea will bring blood to the surface and warm cold hands and feet.

GINKGO *(Ginkgo biloba)*

Parts Used: Leaves, seeds

Properties: Gingko leaves are a circulatory stimulant. They increase blood flow to the brain, enhance energy, improve peripheral circulation to the hands and feet, and more.

GLYCERIN

Properties: Humectant or moisturizing agent found in vegetable and animal fats that is often used in moisturizing creams and lotions; also improves spreadability. It attracts water from the surrounding air as well as from the body's tissues but is not easily absorbed, and will keep the skin surface moist as long as there is sufficient moisture in the air. In a dry climate, glycerin may defeat its purpose as a skin moisturizer by drying out the upper skin layer, and if 100 percent glycerin were applied as a humectant, it could draw moisture from already dry skin. However, since the concentration of glycerin in creams and lotions is usually never more than 50 percent, glycerin can be considered a beneficial ingredient.

GOLDENSEAL *(Hydrastis canadensis)*

Parts Used: Dried rhizome and roots
Properties: Antiseptic, anti-inflammatory, and antimicrobial; tincture is used to bathe irritated skin inflammations, eczema, and measles.
Caution: Not recommended for use during pregnancy, by nursing mothers, or by those with high blood pressure.

GRAPEFRUIT *(Citrus x paradisi)*

Parts Used: Fruit, juice, essential oil
Properties: Astringent, antiseptic, diuretic, cleansing, and tonic to the body.

GUM PLANT *(Grindelia camporum)*

Also Known As: Gumweed, grindelia
Parts Used: Flowering tops
Properties: Decoction as a topical wash is an antidote to dermatitis of rhus poisoning (poison ivy, poison oak, or poison sumac).
Caution: Large doses can irritate kidneys.

HAWTHORN TREE *(Crataegus oxyacantha)*

Also Known As: White thorn
Parts Used: Dried flowers, leaves, fruits or berries
Properties: Positive heart restorative; improves circulation in coronary arteries.

HEATH, SPRING *(Erica carnea)*
Parts Used: Needle-like leaves
Properties: Antiseptic, inhibits bacteria.

HENNA *(Lawsonia inermis, L. alba)*
Parts Used: Powdered leaves, flowers
Properties: As a dye for the skin or nails, tinting the hair.

HONEY
Properties: Emollient, humectant, antiseptic, and bacteriostatic; helps skin retain moisture; can be applied to a wound as a cooling analgesic.

HORSETAIL *(Equisetum arvense)*
Also Known As: Shave grass
Parts Used: Stems
Properties: Astringent; a natural source of silica, selenium, and zinc.

JEWELWEED *(Impatiens pallida, I. capensis)*
Also Known As: Spotted-touch-me-not
Parts Used: Whole herb
Properties: Fresh juice of the herb relieves poison ivy rash.

JOJOBA *(Simmondsia chinensis)*
Parts Used: Seeds, extract of the seeds
Properties: Jojoba (ho ho' ba) extract is an unusual wax ester with antioxidant, antimicrobial, anti-inflammatory, and light emollient properties. It is similar in chemistry to human sebum, the skin's natural restorative fluid. Can help to maintain the suppleness of the skin; conditions and softens skin, hair, and scalp; can aid the healing of wounds; can be used alone or as a base for ointments and creams for dry, chapped skin, as a cuticle and nail conditioner, and with aloe for minor burns and sunburn. Jojoba has few impurities; contains no resins, tars, or alkaloids; and is non-toxic and non-allergenic.

KAOLIN CLAY

Properties: A soft, white clay that draws oils and impurities from the skin.

LAVENDER (*Lavandula* spp.)

Parts Used: Flowers, essential oil
Properties: Pleasant antiseptic, antidepressive, and antimicrobial; calming effect to relieve stress; essential oil can be used externally for aching muscles and to help prevent scarring.
Caution: Avoid during first trimester of pregnancy; not recommended for those with very low blood pressure.

LEMON (*Citrus limon*)

Parts Used: Juice, pulp, rind, essential oil
Properties: Astringent, bleaching, disinfectant; scent is stimulating and refreshing; anti-inflammatory.
Caution: Do not use essential oil in strong sunlight or on sensitive skin.

LEMONGRASS (*Cymbopogon citratus*)

Parts Used: Grass, essential oil
Properties: Refreshing, lemon-like tonic; antiseptic, antidepressant, and astringent.
Caution: Avoid during pregnancy, and do not use on sensitive skin.

LIME (*Tilia* spp.)

Also Known As: Linden tree
Parts Used: Flowers, essential oil
Properties: Nervine, diuretic, tonic; reduces nervous tension; calming; can be a soothing and softening agent in skin-care products.

LINSEED

See Flax.

LOVAGE (*Levisticum officinale*)

Parts Used: Root, leaves, fruit or seeds, stem
Properties: Mild antibiotic, diaphoretic, carminative, aromatic flavoring.

MEADOWSWEET (*Filipendula ulmaria*)

Parts Used: Leaves and stems

Properties: Offers symptomatic relief of indigestion and is often used as an antacid; contains salicylic acid, the precursor of aspirin, and can be used in a tea as an anti-inflammatory and anticoagulant.

MILK, BUTTERMILK, AND CREAM

Properties: Can be used as a skin cleanser and as an emollient in creams and lotions.

MINT (*Mentha* spp.)

Parts Used: Leaves, essential oil

Properties: Stimulant, carminative, antispasmodic, diaphoretic; relieves stomach complaints; can be used for flavoring.

MYRRH (*Commiphora molmol*)

Parts Used: Gum resin, volatile oil

Properties: Antifungal, antibacterial, antiviral agent; antiseptic, cooling, and tonic; good for wounds that refuse to heal, boils, and abscesses.

NETTLE (*Urtica dioica*)

Also Known As: Stinging nettle

Parts Used: Young tops, leaves, juice, seeds

Properties: Rich in vitamin C, calcium, iron, and silica; antiseptic, astringent, mild diuretic, vasodilator, and circulatory stimulant; eliminates uric acid from the body; can be used to treat chronic skin diseases. (An antidote to nettle sting is juice of the dock plant, mint, or sage leaves.)

OATS, OAT STRAW (*Avena sativa*)

Parts Used: Oatmeal or oat bran, seeds, or grains

Properties: Exfoliant and emollient for chapped hands, eczema, and irritated, dry, or itching skin; source of vitamin E, proteins, zinc, iron, and manganese.

OLIVE *(Olea europaea)*

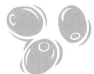

Parts Used: Oil of the fruit, leaves

Properties: Emollient, demulcent, laxative; source of linoleic acid; cold-pressed oil is used in salves for muscle pains; leaves in tea are astringent and antiseptic; may lower blood sugar in diabetes and dilate coronary arteries to improve blood circulation.

ONION *(Allium cepa)*

Parts Used: Bulb

Properties: Antiseptic, antibacterial, anti-inflammatory, and diuretic; rich in vitamins B_1, B_2, and C; stimulates the heart and reduces blood sugar.

ORANGE *(Citrus aurantium)*

Parts Used: Fruit, flowers, rind

Properties: Essential oil of sweet orange blossoms, called *neroli,* has antiseptic, antidepressant, and tonic properties and is a perfect choice for sensitive skin. Essential oil of the leaves and young shoots of the orange, called *oil of petitgrain,* is a natural skin toner and stimulant but may be a bit harsh for sensitive skin.

PAPAYA *(Carica papaya)*

Parts Used: Fruit, juice, leaves

Properties: Juice and fruit of the fresh plant can be used for wounds that refuse to heal and to remove freckles; contains papain, an enzyme that can improve digestion of proteins; leaves may be used as a substitute for soap.

PARAFFIN

Properties: A non-absorbent, odorless, tasteless, colorless or white protective dressing made from a purified mixture of hydrocarbons obtained from petroleum.

PARSLEY *(Petroselinum crispum)*

Parts Used: Leaves, stems

Properties: Antimicrobial, cleansing, and diuretic; rich in potassium, calcium, and silica; may strengthen nails and skin; reduces smell of garlic and onions on breath and hands.

Caution: Not recommended in large doses during pregnancy or by those with kidney inflammation.

PATCHOULI (*Pogostemon patchouli*)
Parts Used: Whole herb, essential oil
Properties: Anti-inflammatory, antiseptic, astringent; cell regenerator for dermatitis, eczema, and aging skin; essential oil has a pungent, earthy scent.

PINEAPPLE (*Ananas comosus*)
Parts Used: Juice, fruit
Properties: Anti-inflammatory; gargle for sore throat.

PLANTAIN (*Plantago major, P. lanceolata*)
Parts Used: Leaves, roots, seeds
Properties: Astringent, demulcent, antiallergy; tones and heals the skin; can reduce body heat; crushed leaves can reduce the swelling of bee stings.

RASPBERRY (*Rubus idaeus*)
Parts Used: Fruit, leaves
Properties: Astringent and stimulant; can be used as a wash for wounds and external skin ulcers.

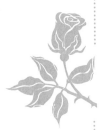

ROSE, OTTO OF (*Rosa damascena*)
Parts Used: Essential oil from the flower
Properties: Astringent, tonic, antiseptic, anti-inflammatory; promotes the formation of new skin cells; especially useful for dry, sensitive, aging skin.
Caution: Limit use during pregnancy.

ROSEMARY (*Rosmarinus officinalis*)
Parts Used: Leaves and stems
Properties: Antispasmodic, rubefacient, and fragrant stimulant; can be used in a liniment to treat painful joints and stiff muscles. In ancient times, rosemary had a reputation for strengthening the memory.

SAGE (*Salvia officinalis*)
Parts Used: Leaves, whole herb
Properties: Astringent and stimulant; used to treat joint pain.
Caution: Not recommended in large doses during pregnancy or by those with high blood pressure or epilepsy.

ST.-JOHN'S-WORT *(Hypericum perforatum)*
Parts Used: Flowers and herb tops
Properties: Alterative, nervine, anti-inflammatory, antidepressant; noted for its ability to relieve pain; especially helpful in injuries to areas rich in nerves, such as fingertips or foot soles.

SEA SALT
Properties: Rich in minerals; circulatory stimulant in a scrub; can remove dead surface skin cells and dirt.
Caution: May burn broken skin.

SEAWEED *(Laminaria digitata)*
Also Known As: Kelp
Parts Used: Seaweed flakes and powder
Properties: Emollient; rich in vitamins and minerals.

SHEA BUTTER *(Botyrospermum parkii)*
Also Known As: Karite butter
Properties: Can be added to moisturizers for the reduction of wrinkles and to creams for sore muscles, rheumatism, burns, and light wounds; antioxidant with a high linoleic acid content; good for dry or irritated skin, sunburn, chapping; offers skin protection against ultraviolet rays; increases capillary circulation; good for sensitive skin.

SORREL *(Rumex acetosa)*
Parts Used: Leaves
Properties: Alterative, diuretic, refrigerant; leaves may help to lighten skin spots of aging.

SWEDISH BITTERS
Parts Used: A combination of 11 traditional bitter herbs macerated in alcohol to form a tincture: aloe (or gentian or wormwood), manna, myrrh, saffron, senna leaves, camphor, rhubarb root, zedoary root, venetian theriac, blessed thistle root, and angelica root.
Properties: Liver stimulant and detoxifier.
Caution: Not recommended for use during pregnancy or by nursing mothers or those with a history of intestinal obstruction.

SWEET FERN *(Comptonia peregrina)*
Parts Used: Leaves
Properties: A wash, bath, or tea of sweet fern leaves is soothing to irritated skin, especially skin that has been exposed to poison ivy.

TEA TREE *(Melaleuca alternifolia)*
Parts Used: Essential oil
Properties: Antifungal, antibacterial, tissue cleanser; a 10% solution of the essential oil is a safe external antiseptic for skin diseases, fungal infections, and wounds.

VALERIAN *(Valeriana officinalis)*
Parts Used: Root or rhizome
Properties: A natural relaxant, calming, sedative, mild pain reliever.

VERVAIN *(Verbena officinalis)*
Parts Used: Leaves, flowering tops
Properties: Astringent and vulnerary; can be used in a poultice to treat rheumatism.
Caution: Not recommended for use during pregnancy.

VIOLET, SWEET *(Viola odorata)*
Parts Used: Flowers and leaves
Properties: Mild analgesic and antiseptic; used in teas and compresses.

VITAMIN E OIL
Also Known As: Natural d-alpha tocopherol (other forms are synthetic)
Properties: A natural preservative; discourages scarring, encourages healing of wounds.

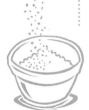

WHEAT GERM *(Triticum aestivum)*
Parts Used: Germ of the wheat
Properties: Antioxidant and emollient; rich in vitamin E.

From: _____
_____
_____

BUSINESS REPLY MAIL

FIRST-CLASS MAIL   PERMIT NO. 2   POWNAL VT

POSTAGE WILL BE PAID BY ADDRESSEE

STOREY'S BOOKS FOR COUNTRY LIVING
STOREY COMMUNICATIONS INC
RR1 BOX 105
POWNAL VT 05261-9988

We'd love your thoughts . . .

Your reactions, criticisms, things you did or didn't like about this Storey Book. Please use space below (or write a letter if you'd prefer
— even send photos!) telling how you've made use of the information . . . how you've put it to work . . . the more details the better!

Thanks in advance for your help in building our library of good Storey Books.

Book Title: _____

Purchased From: _____

Pamela B. Art
Publisher, Storey Books

Comments:

_____

_____

_____

_____

_____

Your Name: _____

Mailing Address: _____

E-mail Address: _____

☐ Please check here if you'd like our latest Storey's Books for Country Living Catalog.

☐ You have my permission to quote from my comments and use these quotations in ads, brochures, mail, and other promotions used
to market Storey Books.

Signed _____ Date _____

e-mail=feedback@storey.com   www.storey.com   PRINTED IN THE USA   4/98

WHEY CONCENTRATE
Properties: Whey concentrate is the thin serum remaining after the curd and cream have been removed from milk. Combined with lactic acid as a homeopathic treatment for eczema.

WILLOW *(Salix alba)*
Parts Used: Dried bark
Properties: Antiseptic; helps to reduce fever; source of salicylic acid (a forerunner of aspirin) and used as a mild painkiller and to reduce inflammatory states of rheumatoid arthritis and painful muscles and joints.

WINTERGREEN *(Gaultheria procumbens)*
Also Known As: Teaberry
Parts Used: Leaves
Properties: Anti-inflammatory, mild analgesic, and diuretic; can be used in a tea or liniment to treat inflammation of the muscles and joints, and rheumatoid arthritis.

WITCH HAZEL *(Hamamelis virginiana)*
Parts Used: Bark, leaves
Properties: Astringent and anti-inflammatory; skin healing; contains bioflavonoids, which can protect capillaries made fragile by steroid therapy.

XANTHAN
Parts Used: Powder
Properties: An enzyme modified from corn starch that breaks into a natural gum; used as a thickener in preparations.

YARROW *(Achillea millefolium)*
Parts Used: Whole herb
Properties: Styptic, vulnerary, and diaphoretic; can be used in a bath to lessen pain, inflammation, and heal wounds; can aid in lowering temperature in the early stages of fever or flu.

YOGURT
Properties: Mildly astringent; rich in B-complex vitamins; contains helpful bacteria that act to restore normal chemical balance to the intestines and aid the body's digestive system.

APPENDIX B:
Basic Equipment and Tools

Most herbal remedies won't require more than the supplies that you normally find in your kitchen. However, I recommend that you try to accumulate a separate set of measuring and stirring tools, bowls, grinders, pots, and more to be set aside just for making herbal blends and treatments. You may not be convinced of the value of this suggestion to start, but wait until you find hard little seeds turning up in your culinary recipes, or your favorite pot overlaid with beeswax or retaining a permanent stain from a natural plant dye.

Here's a list of basic provisions:

COOKING TIP

Be sure that all of your cookware for making herbal remedies is made of nonreactive materials such as glass, enamel, or stainless steel, and not reactive metals such as copper or aluminum.

- All-purpose mixing bowls in a variety of sizes
- Coffee grinder
- Cutting board
- Double boiler
- Funnels
- Glass eyedropper
- Grater
- Heavy-duty plastic zip-seal storage bags
- Ice cube trays
- Jars with screw-top lids, preferably of tinted glass
- Kitchen or garden shears
- Kitchen scale
- Labels and marking pens
- Measuring cups with metric and imperial measurements
- Measuring spoons
- Mortar and pestle
- Multispeed blender or food processor
- Nonreactive pots and saucepans with lids
- Sieves: fine-mesh cheesecloth, unbleached muslin, paper coffee filters, nylon or stainless steel mesh
- Utensils: paring knife, ladle, wooden mallet, vegetable peeler, rolling pin, spatula, wooden spoons, whisk

APPENDIX C:
Terms and Techniques for Preparing Natural Remedies

There are many delivery systems for applying herbal and natural treatments. Most of these methods are quite simple to prepare and have been used for centuries by everyday folks for healing or cosmetic purposes. What follows is a description of some of the most common terms and techniques.

Medicinal Herbs vs. Herbal Medicine

Many herbs in their natural state have antibacterial, antiviral, diuretic, alterative, and/or stimulant properties, and are often called medicinal herbs. These herbs contain groups of powerful constituents, including nutrients, that have been used by cultures across the world to improve wellness. Many of these potent herbs have also been studied extensively by scientists and chemists worldwide, and their medicinal value has been proven time and time again.

Herbal medicine, also known as phytotherapeutic medicine, uses medicinal herbs (and other healing plants that might not qualify as "herbs") to strengthen immune reserves, invigorate the body, and help the body fight infection and disease.

Herbal Infusions

An herbal infusion, also known as an herbal tea, is a simple steeping process that draws out the beneficial properties of herbs into a liquid that can then be drunk as a tea or applied as a wash or soak. Herbal infusions can be prepared with both hot and cold liquid.

One way to prepare an infusion is to pour hot or cold liquid (usually water, juice, or vinegar) over the crushed, ground, or chopped herb and allow to steep, covered, for ten to twenty minutes (sometimes longer for cold infusions). Then strain the infused liquid. A standard infusion is usually 1 ounce (30 g) dried herb (or 3 ounces [90 g] fresh herb) to 2 cups (500 ml) of liquid.

For remedy purposes, the standard adult dosage for drinking an infusion as an herbal tea is one-half cup, three times a day. An infusion can also be used as a wash or soak to bathe irritated or inflamed skin or wounds. Carefully wash the affected area, from the center outward, with the infused liquid, or lightly mist the liquid onto the affected area with an atomizer.

Leftover infused liquid is best stored in a labeled container in a cool place, and should be used within a day or two of preparation.

Infused Oils

Infused oils are pungent, aromatic infusions of herbs in oil applied externally or used as ingredients in creams or salves. Olive oil is frequently the oil of choice, but you can use any variety of cold-pressed oil. As with herbal teas, there is both a hot and a cold method of infusing herbs in oil. Store the oils in a cool, dark location. They will keep for one year.

Cold Oil Infusion. Fill a jar to the brim with slightly bruised herb material. Cover with cold-pressed oil. Seal with a screw-type lid and let sit in a sunny window (or in a paperbag in a sunny window — some herbs lose potency when exposed to the sun's rays) for two to four weeks. Then pour the infused oil through a fine-mesh cheesecloth, being sure to press all of the oil through the cloth. Strain twice if necessary to make sure that all of the herb material is removed. Then discard the herb material.

You can stop here or add new herbs to the jar, refilling with the once-infused oil and repeating the infusion process.

Hot Oil Infusion. In a double boiler, combine the bruised herb and cold-pressed oil according to each recipe's guidelines. Heat gently for at least three hours. Then strain the mixture through a fine-mesh cheesecloth, paper coffee filter, or wine press into a container. Strain a second time if necessary. Using a funnel, pour the oil into airtight dark glass bottles and seal.

Essential Oils

Have you ever peeled an orange and inhaled its essence? If so, then you've been introduced to the world of essential oils. These oils are expressed or distilled from the leaves, stems, bark, flowers, fruits, and roots of many kinds of plants. They are highly concentrated, volatile, and evaporate quickly when exposed to the air or heat. They are also very potent and most often need to be diluted in a carrier oil or dosed in individual drops. Think of essential oils as being 100 times more concentrated than a fresh herb.

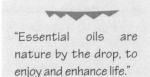

"Essential oils are nature by the drop, to enjoy and enhance life."

— Colleen K. Dodt
The Essential Oils Book

Essential oils are costly, as it can take hundreds or even thousands of pounds of plant material to produce an ounce of essential oil. Steam distillation is one of the most common methods of extraction. Steam is forced into a vat containing the plant material. The intense heat from the steam splits the plant's oil glands, releasing the precious oil. A cold water bath then allows the oil to be collected and bottled.

Essential oils have many uses. Many have antiseptic and anti-inflammatory properties, including bergamot, clary sage, geranium, grapefruit, lavender, lemon, peppermint, rosemary, and tea tree. They are often used in aromatherapy, natural healing remedies, and natural cosmetics.

Compresses

A compress is simply a cloth soaked in a hot herbal infusion that is then applied to the affected area.

Poultices

A poultice is similar to a compress except that plant or herb material is applied directly to the skin, rather than the liquid infusion from which the plant material has been strained, and the cloth is wrapped around the affected area. The plant or herb can be chopped, bruised, boiled, or prepared as a paste with water, honey, or oil. Poultices are commonly used to relieve the pain, swelling, and skin irritation resulting from bruises, sprains, wounds, and skin ulcers.

Decoctions

A decoction is the process of extracting the active components from the hard, woody parts of plants, such as twigs, bark, roots, seeds, and some berries. The woody material is placed in a non-reactive pot, covered with water or another liquid, and boiled for up to an hour (until the liquid volume has been reduced to about one-third). The liquid is then strained or filtered.

Decoctions should be used within one day and stored between uses in a cool place.

Tinctures

A tincture is similar to an herbal infusion, but the liquid in which the herb is steeped is not water but a dilution of alcohol, glycerin, or vinegar and water. The steeping usually takes place at room temperature. A tincture is designed to first draw out and then preserve a plant's active medicinal components. A single dosage prescribed for a tincture may range from a few drops to a couple of teaspoons. Tinctures will keep for up to two years, and should be stored in a cool, dark place.

Creams, Lotions, and Ointments

An **herbal cream** is an emulsion containing herbally infused water and fats or oils that softens and blends with (penetrates) the skin.

An **herbal lotion** is a water and/or tincture-based mixture that can be applied as a cooling remedy to soothe bothered skin.

An **herbal ointment** or **salve** is a semi-solid preparation of medicinal herbs in a variety of non-aqueous bases, such as olive oil, beeswax, or coconut oil, that does not blend with the skin but forms a separate layer over it. It contains only oils or fats and no water, and is used to protect, nourish, or treat sensitive, injured, or thin skin.

Herbal creams, lotions, and ointments can last up to several months if natural preservatives, such as essential oils or tincture of benzoin, are added. They should be kept in a cool location.

Standardized Extracts

A standardized extract is a laboratory preparation of a plant that has been purified and documented to show a consistent and specific concentration of that plant's active components. This assures that each time you take a standardized extract, you can be certain that the proper plant is in the formula and that the effect will be the same or similiar to the previous dose. However, opponents of laboratory standardization feel that the plant and preparations made with it should be kept as close to the natural state of the plant as possible in order to benefit from the total synergy of all of the plant's medicinal actions. The best method is still up for grabs!

Common Cosmetic and Medicinal Terms

These brief definitions will help you understand some of the benefits and applications of the herbs and natural ingredients included in *Natural Hand Care*.

Adaptogen: A substance that helps the body adapt to a new stress by stimulating the body's immune mechanism.

Alterative: Restores the normal functions of a body organ or system.

Analgesic: Relieves pain.

Antiallergy: Reduces allergic reactions and their symptoms.

Antibacterial: Effective against bacteria.

Anti-inflammatory: Works with the body to help reduce swelling and return the tissue to its normal state.

Antimicrobial: Inhibits or destroys microorganisms.

Antioxidant: A compound that protects the body against free-radical activity (oxidants that may have a harmful effect on the lining of blood vessels and other tissues).

Antiseptic: Destroys or inhibits the growth of microorganisms and controls infection.

Antispasmodic: Relieves or prevents muscular cramps or spasms and associated mild pain.

Antiviral: Weakens or destroys viruses.

Astringent: Constricts blood vessels and tissues to reduce secretion and excretion.

Bacteriostatic: Inhibits the growth or multiplication of bacteria.

Bitter: Stimulates appetite and aids in digestion.

Carminative: Relieves flatulence and gastric discomfort.

Compress: External application of an herbal combination to reduce inflammation and pain or soften tissues.

Decoction: Extract of active ingredients from barks, roots, or woody parts of a plant by simmering these materials in water for a period of time and straining the preparation.

Demulcent: Protects and soothes inflamed or irritable surfaces.

Diaphoretic: Increases perspiration.

Diuretic: Helps the body to excrete excess fluid as urine from the kidneys.

Emollient: Lubricates, softens, or soothes skin tissue.

Emulsifier: Used to produce an emulsion by joining oil and water, two ingredients that would normally not mix.

Emulsion: A preparation where oil is suspended in water with the addition of an emulsifier; a convenient way of applying oils to penetrate the skin.

Expectorant: Promotes loosening and ejection of phlegm through coughing from upper respiratory tract.

Humectant: Attracts and promotes retention of moisture; in cosmetics, controls the moisture exchange between the skin, the product, and the air.

Infusion: An herbal tea.

Menstruum: A solvent medium to carry the herbal ingredients.

Mucilage: A slimy or adhesive paste used to give a suitable consistency or form to a remedy.

Nervine: Affects the nervous system; may be stimulating or relaxing.

Neuralgia: Pain radiating along the course of a nerve.

Poultice: A soft, moist mass applied hot to the body's surface as a healing technique.

Rubefacient: Draws a rich blood supply to the skin's surface, increasing heat in and reddening the tissues.

Stimulant: Increases activity of the body's circulatory system, organs, and/or energy.

Styptic: Stops external bleeding.

Tonic: Restoring, invigorating, and toning for specific muscles, tissues, or organs, or the entire body.

Vasoconstrictor: Constricts blood vessels, decreasing diameter.

Vasodilator: Dilates or relaxes blood vessels, increasing diameter.

Vulnerary: Promotes healing of wounds.

READING LIST

Ackerman, Diane. *The Natural History of the Senses.* New York: Random House, 1990.

Balin, Arthur K., M.D., Ph.D., and Loretta Pratt Balin, M.D. *The Life of the Skin.* New York: Bantam Books, 1997.

Bark, Joseph P., M.D. *Skin Secrets.* New York: McGraw-Hill, 1987.

_____.*Your Skin: An Owner's Guide.* Englewood Cliffs, NJ: Prentice-Hall, 1995.

Bartram, Thomas. *Encyclopedia of Herbal Medicine.* Dorset, England: Grace Publishers, 1995.

*Butler, Sharon J. *Conquering Carpal Tunnel Syndrome and Other Repetitive Strain Injuries.* Oakland, CA: New Harbinger Publications, 1996.

Callan, Annette, ed. *Skin Wise: A Guide to Healthy Skin for Women.* Melbourne: Oxford University Press, 1996.

*Cox, Janice. *Natural Beauty at Home.* New York: Henry Holt and Co., 1995.

*Crouch, Tammy, and Michael Madden, D.C. *Carpal Tunnel Syndrome and Overuse Injuries: Prevention, Treatment, and Recovery.* Berkeley, CA: North Atlantic Books, 1992.

Cummins, Harold, and Charles Midlo. *Finger Prints, Palms and Soles.* New York: Dover Publications, 1961.

*Dinsdale, Margaret. *Skin Deep: Natural Recipes for Healthy Skin and Hair.* Ontario: Camden House Publishing, 1994.

Donsky, Howard. *Beauty Is Skin Deep.* Emmaus, PA: Rodale Press, 1985.

*Duke, James A., Ph.D. *The Green Pharmacy.* Emmaus, PA: Rodale Press, 1997.

Dunne, Lavon J. *Nutrition Almanac.* 3rd ed. New York: McGraw-Hill Publishing Co., 1990.

Editors of *Prevention*® Magazine. *The Complete Book of Vitamins and Minerals for Health.* Emmaus, PA: Rodale Press, 1988.

Frawley, David, M.D. *Ayurvedic Healing: A Comprehensive Guide.* Salt Lake City: Passage Press, 1989.

*Gach, Michael Reed. *Arthritis Relief at Your Fingertips.* New York: Warner Books, 1989.

"The History of Nail Care." *Nails.* February 1993.

Holick, Michael F. "Vitamin D Deficiency, The Silent Epidemic." *Nutrition Action Health Letter.* October 1997, 1–6.

Janson, Michael, M.D. *The Vitamin Revolution in Health Care.* Greenville, NH: Arcadia Press, 1996.

Kaufmann, Klaus. *Silica: The Forgotten Nutrient.* New York: Alive Books, 1993.

Klein, Arnold W., M.D., J.H. Sternberg, M.D., and Paul Bernstein, M.D. *The Skin Book.* New York: Collier Books, 1980.

Lerner, Marguerite Rush, M.D. *Horns, Hoofs, Nails.* Minneapolis: Lerner Publications Co., 1966.

*Lorig, Kate, R.N., Ph.D., and James Fries, M.D. *The Arthritis Helpbook.* Reading, MA: Addison-Wesley Publishing Co., 1986.

Marchetti, Albert. *Common Cures for Common Ailments.* New York: Stein and Day Publishers, 1979.

Mességué, Maurice. *Of Men and Plants: The Autobiography of the World's Most Famous Plant Healer.* New York: MacMillan & Co., 1973.

Meyer, Clarence. *American Folk Medicine.* New York: Thomas Y. Crowell Co., 1973.

Milady's Standard Textbook of Cosmetology. Albany, NY: Milady Publishing Co., 1995.

*Montgomery, Kate. *Carpal Tunnel Syndrome.* San Diego, CA: Sports Touch Publishing, 1994.

"The Nail Doctor." *Nails.* December, 1997.

Norton, Lawrence A., M.D. "What Does the White Nail Mean?" *Dermatology Digest.* January 1969, 51–56.

*Ody, Penelope. *The Complete Medicinal Herbal.* London: Dorling Kindersley, 1993.

Revesz, Geza. *The Human Hand: A Psychological Study.* London, Routledge and Paul, 1958.

Schoen, Linda A., and Paul Lazar, M.D. *The Look You Like.* New York: Marcel Dekker, 1990.

*Smeh, Nikolaus J. *Creating Your Own Cosmetics — Naturally.* Garrisonville, VA: Alliance Publishing Co., 1995.

Sorell, Walter. *The Story of the Human Hand.* New York: Bobbs-Merrill Co., 1967.

Strehlow, Wighard, and Gottfried Hertzka, M.D. *Hildegard of Bingen's Medicine.* Santa Fe: Bear & Co., 1988.

Tabori, Paul. *The Book of the Hand: A Compendium of Fact and Legend Since the Dawn of History.* Philadelphia: Chilton Co., 1962.

Tyler, Varro E., Ph.D. *The Honest Herbal.* 3rd ed. New York: Haworth Press, 1993.

*Vogel, Alfred, et al. *The Nature Doctor: A Manual of Traditional and Complementary Medicine.* New Canaan, CT: Keats Publishing, 1991.

Weiss, Rudolf F., M.D. *Herbal Medicine.* Translated by A.R. Meuss. Beaconsfield, England: Beaconsfield Publishers, Ltd., 1988.

Wilkerson, James A., ed. *Hypothermia, Frostbite, and Other Cold Injuries.* Seattle: The Mountaineers, 1986.

Woodbury, William A. *Beauty Culture.* New York: G.W. Dillingham Co., 1910.

*A practical, how-to guide

RESORCES

RESEARCH INFORMATION ON MEDICINAL HERBS

American Botanical Council
P.O. Box 201660
Austin, TX 78720
(512) 331-8868
Fax: (512) 331-1924
Web site: www.herbalgram.org
Email: abc@herbalgram.org

American Herb Association
P.O. Box 1673
Nevada City, CA 95959-1673
(530) 265-9552
Fax: (530) 274-3140

Herb Research Foundation
1007 Pearl Street, Suite 200
Boulder, CO 80302
(303) 449-2265
Fax: (303) 449-7849
Web site: www.herbs.org

United Plant Savers
P.O. Box 420
East Barre, VT 05649
(802) 476-3722
Web site: www.plantsavers.org
Replant endangered or threatened plant species into the environment for nonharvestable purposes

MAIL–ORDER SUPPLIERS FOR HERBS AND NATURAL PRODUCTS

Aromatherapy International
3319 River Pines Road
Ann Arbor, MI 48103
(800) 722-4377
Fax: (734) 741-7109
Quality essential oils

Aubrey Organics
4419 N. Manhattan Avenue
Tampa, FL 33614
(813) 877-4186
A variety of natural preparations, including organic aloe vera gel, evening primrose oil, and more

California Olive Oil Corp.
134 Canal Street
Salem, MA 01970
(978) 745-7840
Fax: (978) 744-3492
A variety of oils, including almond oil, avocado oil, coconut oil, and olive oil

Cedar Spring Herb Farm
159 Long Pond Drive
Harwich, MA 02645
(508) 771-4372
A variety of herbs and herbal preparations, including Caramel Cubes and
dandelion blossom salve

Cosmetic Supply Company
28 Hulvey Drive
Stafford, VA 22554
(540) 659-2097
Fax: (540) 659-4497
Alginate, xanthan, papaya enzyme,
vitamin C powders; Germaben II;
phospholipids; oils; and more

Dry Creek Herb Farm
13935 Dry Creek Road
Auburn, CA 95602
(916) 878-2441
A variety of organic and wildcrafted
herbs and herbal preparations

Eclectic Institute
14385 S.E. Lusted Road
Sandy, OR 97055
(800) 332-4372
Fax: (503) 668-3227
Freeze-dried herbs and vitamins

Frontier Cooperative Herbs
3021 78th Street
P.O. Box 299
Norway, IA 52318
(800) 669-3275
Web site: www.frontierherb.com
Organic and wildcrafted bulk herbs
and herbal products; free catalog

Gaia Herbs
108 Island Ford Road
Bravard, NC 28712
(800) 831-7780
Herbs, Siberian ginseng tonic,
Swedish bitters, and more

**Gold Mine Natural Food Com-
pany**
3419 Hancock Street
San Diego, CA 92110-4307
(800) 475-3663
Ceramic mortar and pestle

Healing Spirits Herb Farm
Matthias and Andrea Reisen
9198 State Route 415
Avoca, NY 14809
(607) 566-2701
A small, family-owned business
that offers apprenticeships;
organic and wildcrafted herbs such
as burdock seed, calendula, dandelion, horsetail, and red clover;
beeswax; and more

Heel/BHI
11600 Cochiti Road, SE
Albuquerque NM 87123-3376
(800) 621-7644
Homeopathic Traumeel® ointment
used for carpal tunnel syndrome

Herbal Earth
P.O. Box 56
Epsom, NH 03234
(603) 463-7251
Fax: (603) 463-7230
Herbs, creams, oils, salves,
newsletter

Herbs 'n Honey
281 Monson Road
Stafford Springs, CT 06076
(860) 684-0551
Beeswax, honey ointment, cleansing grains, and more

Indiana Botanic Gardens
P.O. Box 5
Hammond, IN 46325-0005
(800) 644-8327
Bulk herbs for teas and skin remedies; free catalog

Jean's Greens
R.R. 1, Box 55J
Hale Road
Rensslaerville, NY 12147
(888) 845-8327
Fax: (315) 845-6501
Herbal teas, herbs and spices, herbal supplies; free catalog

Lavender Lane
7337 #1 Roseville Road
Sacramento, CA 95842
(888) 593-4400
Fax: (916) 339-0842
Hard-to-find herbs and herbalware (such as alkanet root, beeswax pearls, oils, and bottles); free catalog

Liberty Natural Products
8120 SE Stark Street
Portland, OR 97215
(503) 256-1227
Offers a variety of herbal extracts, essential oils, and natural products; catalog available

Max Emanual Apotheke
Lydia Meinhold
Belgradstrasse 21
Munich, Germany 80796
Wermutsalbe

Mori-Nu
2050 West 190th Street, Suite 110
Torrance, CA 90504
(310) 787-0200
Web site: www.morinu.com
"Silken" Tofu

Mountain Rose Herbs
20818 High Street
North San Juan, CA 95960
(800) 879-3337
Fax: (916) 292-9138
Web site:
www.botanical.com/mtrose
Organically grown herbs, cosmetic ingredients, bottles; catalog available

NutriBiotic
133 Copeland Street
Petaluma, CA 94952
(707) 769-2266
Web site: www.nutriteam.com
Grapefruit extract and many natural products

San Francisco Herb & Natural Food Co.
47444 Kato Road
Fremont, CA 94538
(510) 770-1215
Fax: (510) 770-9021
Large selection of organic and wild-crafted herbs and herbal products

SKS Bottle & Packaging, Inc.
3 Knabner Road
Mechanicville, NY 12118
(518) 899-7488
Fax: (518) 899-7490
Wide selection of bottles and jars
for cosmetic packaging

Tieraona's Herbals
Tieraona Low Dog, M.D.
120 Hermosa SE
Albuquerque, NM 87108
(800) 553-4165
Fax: (505) 232-3162
Herbal preparations such as
arnica cream, calendula cream,
evening primrose cream, and more

Trout Lake Farm
149 Little Mountain Road
Trout Lake, WA 98650
(800) 395-6093
Fax: (509) 395-2645
Trout Lake Farm herbs are kosher
certified, but at this point they
sell their herbs only in quantities
of 10 pounds and more

Vermont Country Store
Apothecary
P.O. Box 3200
Manchester Center, VT 05255-
3200
(802) 362-0405
Fax: (802) 362-0285
Old-time comforts and remedies,
including B & O'R Lotion

Wild Weeds
P.O. Box 88
302 Camp Weott Road
Ferndale, CA 95536
(800) 553-9453
Fax: (800) 836-9453
Handmade herbals, herb seeds,
medicinal herbs and plants (such
as alkanet, myrrh, plantain, and
red clover), herbalist supplies
(such as tight-weave cheesecloth),
and more

RECOMMENDED FIELD GUIDES TO MEDICINAL PLANTS

Edible and Medicinal Plants of the West, Gregory Tilford. Missoula, MT: Mountain Press, 1997.

Edible Wild Plants, Thomas J. Elias and Peter A. Dykeman. New York: Sterling Publishers, 1990.

The Herb Book, John Lust. New York: Bantam Books, 1974.

Peterson's Guide to Medicinal Plants, Steven Foster and James Duke. Boston: Houghton Mifflin, 1990.

Weeds of the West Compendium. Newark, CA: Western Society of Weed Science.

GLOVES AND OTHER HAND PROTECTORS

Burnham Glove Co.
1602 Tennessee Street
P.O. Box 276
Michigan City, IN 46360
(800) 535-2544
Garden, thorn-guard gloves;
adults and children

Carolina Glove Co.
Dept. TR
P.O. Box 820
Newton, NC 28658
(800) 438-6888
Garden and leather gloves

Dome Industries
Handeze Therapeutic Support
Gloves
10 New England Way
Warwick, RI 02886
(800) 279-7456
Gloves to prevent overuse wrist
injuries

Grab On Products
100 North Avery Street
P.O. Box 2276
Walla Walla, WA 99362
(509) 529-9800
Pen, pencil, and tool cushion grips

Guardian Products
P.O. Box 150357
San Rafael, CA 94915-0357
(415) 258-0601
Full-fashioned cotton gloves

Hawkeye Glove Mfg.
516 North 6th Street
P.O. Box 601, Dept. T
Fort Dodge, IA 50501
(800) 426-7535
Leather work gloves and mittens

Intruder Gloves
P.O. Box 136
Rice Lake, WI 54868
(800) 553-5129
Fishing fillet gloves

Jacob Ash Co., Inc.
301 Munson Street
McKees Rock, PA 15136
(800) 245-6111
Fishing and hunting gloves

Jets Glove Manufacturing
7869-T Kensington Court
Brighton, MI 48116
(800) 688-8878
Leather, work, and garden gloves

The John Plant Co.
P.O. Box 527
Ramseur, NC 27316-0527
(800) 334-2711
Cotton and nylon gloves, finger
protectors

Memphis Glove
5321 E. Shelby Drive
Memphis, TN 38118
(901) 795-0672
Leather, cotton, and synthetic
gloves

Seirus Gloves
9076 Carroll Way
San Diego, CA 92121
(800) 447-3787
Ski gloves

Walt Nicke's Garden Talk
36 McLeod Lane
P.O. Box 433
Topsfield, MA 01983
(508) 887-3388
Garden gloves

Williams-Sonoma
Mail Order Department
P.O. Box 7456
San Francisco, CA 94120-7456
(800) 541-2233
Household and garden gloves

Women's Work Gloves
P.O. Box 543
York, ME 03909
(800) 639-2709
Gloves that fit women's hands

RESOURCES FOR LEFTIES

Lefthanded Computer Keyboards Inc.
354 Eisenhower Parkway
Livingston, NJ 07039
(800) 505-3389

Lefthander International
P.O. Box 8249
North Topeka Boulevard
Topeka, KS 66608
(913) 234-2177
Publishes Lefthander magazine

National Association of Left-Handed Golfers
6448 Shawnee Court
Independence, KY 41051
(800) 844-6254
Web site: www.dca.net/golf/
Newsletter, equipment

Southpaw Guitars
5813 Bellaire Boulevard
Houston, TX 77081
(713) 667-5791
Fax: (713) 667-4091

DEAD SEA RESORTS, SPAS, AND SKIN PRODUCTS

Phone: Call the Israel Ministry of Tourism Information Line at (800) 596-1199, and choose option #4.

Internet: For Dead Sea products, try these Internet addresses:

- www.psoriasis.com
  (The Psoriasis Natural Products Center)

- www.olim.co.il
  (Olim Industries of Israel, NA)

- www.ahava.com
  (AHAVA)

ORGANIZATIONS

American Association of Naturopathic Physicians
2366 Eastlake Avenue E., Suite 322
Seattle, WA 98102
(206) 323-7610
Can provide referrals to national network of natural practitioners

The American College of Integrative Medicine
School of Phytotherapy
10401 Montgomery Parkway NE
Albuquerque, NM 87111
(505) 275-0620
Offers a Bachelor of Science degree in herbal medicine

The American Occupational Therapy Association
4720 Montgomery Lane
P.O. Box 31220
Bethesda, MD 20824-1220
(800) 729-2682
Fax: (301) 652-7711
(800) 377-8555 TDD
Booklets on home rehabilitation exercises and carpal tunnel syndrome

American Society of Hand Therapists (ASHT)
401 North Michigan Avenue
Chicago, IL 60611-4267
(312) 321-6866
Fax: (312) 527-6636
Has a database of qualified hand therapists; publishes the Journal of Hand Therapy

International Hand Research Library
100 East Liberty Street
Suite 100
Louisville, KY 40202
(800) 361-9965
Web site: www.handlibrary.org
E-mail: info@handlibrary.com
A not-for-profit library serving as a globally accessible, comprehensive resource library and archives for all scientific, medical, and general information related to the hand

National Institute of Ayurvedic Medicine (NIAM)
584 Milltown Road
Brewster, NY 10509
(888) 246-6426
Fax: (914) 278-8700
Web site: www.niam.com

REHABILITATION CATALOG

Sammons Preston
Enrichments Program
Priority Code C50
P.O. Box 5050
Bolingbrook, IL 60440-9973
(800) 323-5547
In-depth catalog featuring aids for daily living and orthopedic supplies for those with conditions that impact hand movements; source for Palmguard gloves, arthritis elbow supports, ergonomic canes, softouch scissors, thumb and wrist supports, ergonomic pens, and hand-friendly kitchen and garden tools

MANICURE TOOLS

Beatrice Kaye
The Natural Nail Cosmetic Company
12970 San Vicente Boulevard
Los Angeles, CA 90049
(310) 394-3277
Fax: (310) 451-4469
Reasonably priced, well-designed manicure bowl, kit, soaking treatment; cuticle cream; moisturizer; "Push 10," a plastic wand with a correctly formed, right-angle tip for gently pushing back cuticles

E-Nails
Web site: www.gap.com
Produced by The Gap, Ltd., and publicized as the world's first virtual manicure; nail polish with "no wait, no fumes, no acetone."
The web site offers digital displays of the newest nail colors.
1. First, call-up E-nails' virtual hand and select the skin tone closest to your own.
2. Then, choose one of eleven nail color shades and click on a nail.
3. You can wear a different shade on each nail without any chemicals touching your skin!

Flowery Beauty Products
1 Seneca Place
P.O. Box 4008
Greenwich, CT 06830-0008
(800) 545-5247
A company with "grit" appeal; invented the emery board and has enlarged on that product for every kind of fingernail; new products are Purifiles,™ an immersible, sanitizable board to be used against the spread of infection for you and your nail salon; also produces birch wood orange sticks that are thicker than normal and have a protective carnauba wax coating

Tweezerman Beauty Tools
Consumer Services
55 Sea Cliff Avenue
Glen Cove, NY 11542
(800) 645-3340
Web site: www.tweezerman.com
Offers all kinds of tweezers and nail-care tools with a lifetime sharpening guarantee, including Splintertweeze — a needle point splinter remover; tweezers for tick removal; a baby manicure kit with a safe design; baby nail scissors that make it virtually impossible to cut the skin; and Germbuster, an instant hand sanitizer; free catalog

INDEX

Recipe names are in **boldface** type; page references in *italicized* type indicate illustrations.

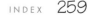

Hives, 118, 146–47, 148
  Amish Cleansing Tea, 146
  Mint Tea Cubes, 147
  Oatmeal Hand Bath, 147
Homeopathy, 66
Honey, 228
  **Almonds, Comfrey, and Honey
    Soothing Ointment,** 136
  Honey Ointment, 211
Horizontal ridges on fingernails, 53,
  55
Horsetail *(Equisetum arvense),* 228
  Horsetail Compress, 141
  Horsetail Nail Bath, 69
  **Horsetail Tea for Brittle
    Nails,** 69
Huan-qi. *See* Astragalus

I

Ice, Compression, Elevation (ICE),
  171
Immune system, 75, 77, 118, 120,
  162
Index finger, 3, *3,* 16
Infections, 55, *55,* 60–64. *See also*
  Fungus infections
Infusions, herbal, 123, 132, 237–38
Injuries. *See also* Overuse injuries
  fingernail, 53, 54
  frostbite, 144–45
  paper cuts, 149
  sprains, 171–72
Iron, 45
Itching skin/hands, 148–49. *See also*
  Allergies; Eczema; Hives

J

Jewelweed *(Impatiens pallida,
    I. capensis),* 150, *150,* 152, 228
  Jewelweed Ice Cubes, 151
Joints
  arthritis, 184–89
  carpal tunnel syndrome, 173–78
  Dupuytren's contracture, 179
  exercises for, 189–90
  Ginger Warming Compress,
    178
  of the hands, 24
  protecting, 166–67

sprains, 171–72
strengthening, 168–71
structure/function of, 164–65,
  165
trigger finger, 180
types of, 166
Jojoba *(Simmondsia chinensis),* 114,
  228

K

Kaolin clay, 229
Karite butter *(Botyrospermum
    parkii),* 233
Keloids, 156–58
Keratin, 21, 48, 51
Kitchen Cabinet Hand Lotion,
  110
Knitbone. *See* Comfrey
Knuckles, cracking, 166

L

Lactic acid, 114
Lactobacillus, 132
Lanolin, 114
Latex allergy, 65
Lavender *(Lavandula* spp.), 132,
  156, 229
  Lavender Flower Wash, 133
  Warm Flower Soak, 61
Left-handedness, 28–29
Lemon *(Citrus limon),* 201, 229
  Lemonade Hands, 107
  Lemon Folk Remedy, 64
  **Mrs. Leyel's Lemon-Egg Skin
    Treatment,** 143
Lemongrass *(Cymbopogon citratus),*
  229
Leopard's bane *(Arnica montana),*
  218
Ligaments, 25, *25,* 26, 165
Lighteners, skin, 136, 201
  Elder Flower Freckle Wash,
    142
  **Mrs. Leyel's Lemon-Egg Skin
    Treatment,** 143
  Tropical Bleaching Lotion,
    202
Lime *(Tilia* spp.), 229
Linden tree *(Tilia* spp.), 229

OTHER STOREY TITLES YOU WILL ENJOY

Natural Foot Care, by Stephanie Tourles. A companion volume to *Natural Hand Care.* Includes herbal recipes, exercises, pedicure instructions, and massage techniques for healthy feet. Includes a chapter on preventing and curing common foot problems. 192 pages. Paperback. ISBN 1-58017-054-4.

The Herbal Body Book: A Natural Approach to Healthier Hair, Skin, and Nails, by Stephanie Tourles. Contains more than 100 recipes to transform common herbs, fruits, and grains into safe, economical, and natural personal care items such as facial scrubs, shampoos, lip balms, and powders. 128 pages. Paperback. ISBN 0-88266-880-3.

The Herbal Home Remedy Book: Simple Recipes for Tinctures, Teas, Salves, Tonics, and Syrups, by Joyce A. Wardwell. Enables the reader to identify and use twenty-five easy-to-find herbs to make simple remedies in the form of teas, tinctures, salves, tonics, vinegars, syrups, and lozenges. Gives hundreds of suggestions for maintaining health and well-being simply, naturally, and inexpensively. Folklore — including Native American legends and stories — provides information on the origins of many herbal medicines. 176 pages. Paperback. ISBN 1-58017-016-1.

The Herbal Home Spa: Naturally Refreshing Wraps, Rubs, Lotions, Masks, Oils, and Scrubs, by Greta Breedlove. Easy-to-make recipes using herbs, fruits, flowers, and essential oils for homemade health and beauty aids that pamper every part of the body from face to feet. Also offers herbal bathing rituals and many massage techniques for treating one's friends to a relaxing spa treatment. 208 pages. Paperback. ISBN 1-58017-005-6.

The Essential Oils Book: Creating Personal Blends for Mind and Body, by Colleen K. Dodt. Discusses the many uses of aromatherapy and its applications in everyday life. Includes simple recipes that anyone can make from ingredients available at health food stores or herb shops. 160 pages. Paperback. ISBN 0-88266-913-3.

Perfumes, Splashes & Colognes: Discovering and Crafting Your Personal Fragrances, by Nancy M. Booth. Profiles basic scent and perfume ingredients, and offers recipes for creating personalized scents or recreating popular perfumes at a fraction of the cost of the original. 176 pages. Paperback. ISBN 0-88266-985-0.

Natural BabyCare: Pure and Soothing Recipes and Techniques for Mothers and Babies, by Colleen K. Dodt. Offers recipes for creating natural personal care items for babies, such as lotions, bath and massage oils, creams, shampoos, and powders. Also features self-care during pregnancy and childbirth. 160 pages. Paperback. ISBN 0-88266-953-2.

These and other Storey books are available at your bookstore, farm store, and garden center, or directly from Storey Books, Schoolhouse Road, Pownal, Vermont 05261, or by calling 1-800-441-5700. Or visit our web site at www.storey.com.